Heart and Emotion:
Ambulatory Monitoring Studies in Everyday Life

Heart and Emotion

Ambulatory Monitoring Studies in Everyday Life

Michael Myrtek

Psychophysiological Research Group,
University of Freiburg i.Br., Germany

Hogrefe & Huber

Library of Congress Cataloging-in-Publication Data

is now available via the Library of Congress Marc Database under the

LC Control Number: 2003116404

National Library of Canada Cataloguing-in-Publication

Myrtek, Michael
Heart and emotion : ambulatory monitoring studies in everyday life / Michael Myrtek.

Includes bibliographical references and index.
ISBN 0-88937-286-1

1. Heart rate monitoring. 2. Emotions--Health aspects. 3. Stress (Physiology) 4. Heart--Psychophysiology. I. Title.

QP113.M97 2004 612.1'71 C2003-907356-4

PUBLISHING OFFICES
USA: Hogrefe & Huber Publishers, 875 Massachusetts Avenue, 7th Floor, Cambridge, MA 02139
Phone (866) 823-4726, Fax (617) 354-6875, E-mail info@hhpub.com
Europe: Hogrefe & Huber Publishers, Rohnsweg 25, D-37085 Göttingen, Germany, Phone +49 551 49609-0, Fax +49 551 49609-88, E-mail hh@hhpub.com

SALES & DISTRIBUTION
USA: Hogrefe & Huber Publishers, Customer Services Department, 30 Amberwood Parkway, Ashland, OH 44805,
Phone (800) 228-3749, Fax (419) 281-6883, E-mail custserv@hhpub.com
Europe: Hogrefe & Huber Publishers, Rohnsweg 25, D-37085 Göttingen, Germany, Phone +49 551 49609-0, Fax +49 551 49609-88, E-mail hh@hhpub.com

OTHER OFFICES
Canada: Hogrefe & Huber Publishers, 1543 Bayview Avenue, Toronto, Ontario M4G 3B5
Switzerland: Hogrefe & Huber Publishers, Länggass-Strasse 76, CH-3000 Bern 9

Hogrefe & Huber Publishers
Incorporated and registered in the State of Washington, USA, and in Göttingen, Lower Saxony, Germany

Printed with the support of the Deutsche Forschungsgemeinschaft

Printed and bound in Germany
ISBN 0-88937-286-1

Preface

> No pen can describe, no words can express, I say, the strange impression which this thing made upon my spirits; I felt something shoot thro' my blood, my heart flutter'd; my head flash'd, and was dizzy, and all within me, as I thought, turn'd about, and much ado I had, not to abandon myself to an excess of passion at the first sight of her, much more when my lips touch'd her face...(Daniel Defoe, 1724, Roxana, p. 342).

Many poets have described the connection between emotional arousal and bodily changes, especially changes in heart rate. There is no doubt – as we all know from our own experience – that, e.g., there is an increase in heart rate during *acute* anxiety. This common observation is surely the main reason for the assumption of a psychosomatic or psychophysiological covariation. In his famous book entitled "Bodily changes in pain, hunger, fear and race," Cannon (1929) described the physiological basis of this emergency reaction.

In everyday life, these strong emotional reactions are rare events. However, as our studies will show the heart reacts to nearly all stimuli throughout the day and even at night. Interestingly, we are not aware of this ongoing activity, with the exception of the above mentioned strong emotional states. The psychosomatic covariation which is so impressive in an acute emotional state is decoupled by this unawareness.

The studies presented in this book were only possible because of the development of a new ambulatory monitoring method. The essential element of this method is the decomposition of heart rate in a physical and a psychological (emotional, mental) component. This is done by the measurement of physical activity and heart rate and the simultaneous comparison of both parameters. Starting point for the development of this method was a clinical research question on the effects of emotional arousal on myocardial functions. Our method, however, is also fruitful for studies on emotions as well as for research in ergonomics.

Chapter 1 of this book deals with some definitions and models which are relevant in the present context. The literature cited is only part of the bulk of literature in this field and only sets an appropriate frame of reference. This Chapter also describes the foundations of our monitoring method. In Chapter 2 basic physiological principles of the nervous control of the heart and the neurophysiology of emotion are briefly described. Chapter 3 is devoted to the description of the monitoring method used in our studies. Because this method is new, information pertaining to the reliability and validity is important. Chapters 4 to 7 are the main chapters of this book containing the results and the discussion of our studies. Especially relevant is Chapter 4 on interoception because these results form a basis for the perception of emotions (Chapter 5) and for the understanding of stress and strain at the workplace (Chapter 6) and during leisure time (Chapter 7). Chapter 8 deals with monitoring during sleep. In the final Chapter 9, a general discussion of all our findings is given.

In the last 15 years, many studies with more than 1,300 subjects were conducted with our *Freiburg Monitoring System* (FMS; Myrtek, Foerster & Brügner, 2001; Myrtek & Foerster, in press). This enormous task is beyond the work of one individual alone. Therefore, the author would like to acknowledge the assistance of many co-workers. My specials thanks to Prof. Dr. J. Fahrenberg, who created the basis for our research group in the 1960s. His helpful and valued comments accompanied our work. He also organized two very fruitful meetings with other researchers in the field of ambulatory monitoring (Fahrenberg & Myrtek, 1996, 2001). My gratitude should also be expressed to G. Brügner (†) who developed the basic algorithms of our monitoring device. F. Foerster has continued his work and created new algorithms for the detection of posture and motion. My thanks to P. Hüttner who developed algorithms for the recording of behavior and subjective state. W. Müller (†) solved many problems concerning the hardware and V. Höppner contributed to the development of hardware components. G. Jansen is acknowledged for her careful data transfer. The doctoral and graduate students who assisted in conducting the experiments are mentioned as co-authors at the appropriate places in the text. My thanks to M. Cheetham for improving the text. Finally, I wish to acknowledge gratefully the financial support of the German Society for the Advancement of Scientific Research (Deutsche Forschungsgemeinschaft, DFG).

Autumn 2003 Michael Myrtek

The reader is advised to read first only the shadowed summaries and Chapter 9.5 Conclusions.

Contents

Chapter 1

Definitions and models

1.1 Emotion

According to James (1892), emotions result from the bodily expression: "My theory, on the contrary is that the *bodily changes follow directly the perception of the exciting fact, and that our feeling of the same changes as they occur* IS *the emotion*" (p. 242). However, James does not describe how the bodily changes are initiated by the perception of the exciting fact (Parkinson, 1988). If this theory were correct, one would have to postulate many different autonomic response patterns to explain the many different emotions. James' theory is called the peripheralist approach and is opposed to the centralist approach proposed by Cannon. According to Cannon (1929) "the responses in the viscera seem too uniform to offer a satisfactory means of distinguishing emotions which are very different in subjective quality" (p. 352). Moreover, visceral changes (with the exception of the heart) are too slow to be a source of emotional feeling. Finally, artificial induction of visceral changes typical of strong emotions by epinephrine does not produce emotions. Cannon argues that activation of central processes in the brain leads to the various symptoms (autonomic responses, motor responses, subjective state) associated with emotion.

As yet no satisfactory definition of what an emotion might be has been given. Plutchik (2003) cites 21 definitions by different authors. Contemporary definitions stress the one or the other aspect proposed by either James or Cannon. The theories by Levenson (1988, 1994) and by Schachter and Singer (1962) are somewhat more closer to James' whereas Pennebaker's view (1982) is more centralistic in pointing out the cognitive aspects. Other authors do not try to define emotion and only list the components involved in an emotional reaction (Lang, 1993; Scherer, 1990, 2000). I hope that our empirical results on the perception of emotions will elucidate the contradictory standpoints.

1.1.1 A look at emotion research

Emotions are an integral part of human life and are of central importance in quite different research questions such as the influence of emotional arousal on clinically important ECG changes (e.g., arrhythmias, ischemic episodes), the degree of emotional work load in comparing differing working places, and the study of emotional arousal producing situations, to mention but a few. However, emotion research has to deal with several problems, the most important of which are the method of emotion induction, the interaction of the different response systems (verbal-cognitive, physiological, behavioral), and the specificity of physiological responses for differing emotions.

The validity of emotion induction is equivocal for both laboratory and field studies. The study of emotional phenomena has been until now typically confined to laboratory situations in which the experimenter tries to elicit different emotional states. As opposed to field studies, subjects in laboratory experiments know that they will be exposed to special situations which may enhance the correlations between physiological activation and self-reported emotional states. On the other hand, field studies also have limitations because they have to rely on self reports of emotion perception. As we will show later, we have to account for subjective hypotheses and schemata as proposed by several authors (Myrtek, 1998a; Pennebaker, 1982; Rimé, Philippot, & Cisamolo, 1990) which distort the perception of an emotion.

A second problem pertains to the interaction of the different response systems. Verbal reports, behavioral responses, and physiological activity are coupled imperfectly (Lang, 1993). Lang (p. 22) states that "it is possible and even usual to generate emotional cognitions without autonomic arousal, aggressive behavior without a hostile motive, or the autonomic and avoidant behavior of fear without insight (proper labeling)." According to Schachter and Singer (1962) physiological changes actually cause the emotion. This emotion perception model assumes that there is activity in different physiological processes which are detected by some higher-order system to generate an emotion report. However, the perception model has been criticized (Reisenzein, 1983).

The third problem deals with the different physiological responses for different emotions. The notion of systematic response profiles associated with various emotions (Levenson, 1988) is still a matter of debate. Levenson (1994) states that the emotions anger, fear, and sadness produce larger increases in heart rate than disgust. The author demonstrated that these differences show consistency across subject populations of different profession, age, culture, and gender. As to happiness, Levenson reports that anger and fear produce larger heart rate accelerations than happiness.

The study of emotional reactions in everyday life relies as yet on self-reported emotional events, mostly assessed by diaries. Naturally, subjects can report only those emotional events they are aware of, leading to the difficult question of to what extent physiological activation of emotional origin is actually perceived. Pennebaker (1982) has shown that emotion perception is not necessarily linked to physiological changes but seems essentially to be a function of cognitive schemas, hypotheses, and so on. Therefore, it would be very important to first detect events with presumably emotionally-induced physiological activation under conditions of daily life and to subsequently acquire time-locked information of the subjective feeling of the individual during such events. Our experience tells us that the method used in our studies is suitable to meet these requirements.

1.1.2 Methods in emotion research

In laboratory experiments dependent variables are activities of the autonomic nervous system (ANS), the somatic nervous system, and self-reports of the emotional state. Several autonomic measures have been used such as heart rate, respiration, and electrodermal activity (e.g., Johnsen, Thayer, & Hugdahl, 1995; Stemmler, 1989). Examples for the measurements in the somatic nervous system are the interpretation of facial expressions (Houle & Feldman, 1991; Wilson, 1991) and the measurement of emotional coactivation of facial muscles by EMG (Dimberg, 1997; Fridlund & Izard, 1983; Jäncke, 1994).

The most important variable in psychophysiological research is heart rate, because heart rate is a sensitive indicator of the arousal of the ANS. Heart rate increases during all emotions, possibly with the exception of disgust (Levenson, 1988), during mental activation, during psychosocial stress, and during many motivational states such as thirst and hunger. However, heart rate increases are also caused to a much larger extent by physical exercise, postural changes, changes in temperature, and changes in altitude, to mention only the most important factors. Therefore, a mere heart rate increase cannot be interpreted as a part of an emotional state without further information. In our field studies, heart rate and physical activity play the most dominant role (see below).

1.1.3 Evolutionary aspects

Cannon (1929) described the increase in "adrenin" and the increase of blood sugar (as a source of muscular energy) following strong emotional experiences. He pointed to the "reflex character" (p. 196) of these reactions and argued that reflexes as a rule are useful responses because they are very quick. The reactions "render the organism more efficient in the physical struggle for existence" (p. 206). Therefore, emotions have a protective function. Levenson (1988) argues that emotions are an efficient mechanism to mobilize and organize disparate response systems to events that pose a threat to survival.

An increase in heart rate is a sign of emotion in humans, mammals, and some other vertebrates, and obviously this is rooted in evolution. Cabanac (1999) was interested in the phylogenesis of emotion and conducted some experiments with rats, lizards, and frogs. In lizards, heart rate increased after 1 minute of gentle handling from 70 bpm (beats/min) to 110 bpm and gradually decreased thereafter in the next five minutes. The same was true for a rat in which heart rate increased from about 360 bpm to 460 bpm in the first minute. The duration of tachycardia was longer in the rat than in the lizards and significant differences to the control period were observed till the 14th minute after handling. No significant differences during handling were observed in frogs.

These findings suggest that emotional stress was present in lizards and absent in frogs. Cabanac argues that emotion is a mental feeling and animals possessing emotion have consciousness. Therefore, it can be assumed that emotion might have emerged phylogenetically in reptiles. Emotion as indicated by emotional tachycardia and emotional fever (elevation of the core temperature by emotional arousal) is present in reptiles, birds, and mammals but not in amphibians and fish.

Another evolutionary aspect is the facial expression of emotional reactions in the context of social behavior. A number of emotions, such as anger, fear, and happiness are manifested as different facial expressions and are obviously inborn (Dimberg, 1988). Human subjects, and primates too, are biologically prepared for emotional communication in a face-to-face interaction. This emotional communication in social interaction is accompanied by the appropriate reactions of the ANS. Aureli, Preston, and de Waal (1999) studied the heart rates of two middle-ranking adult females living in a group of rhesus macaques by heart rate telemetry under natural conditions. The behavior of the subjects and a spoken commentary were videotaped while time markers were inserted in the heart rate data file. Two types of social interactions were investigated, while controlling for the effects of posture and activity of the subjects. The first interaction consisted of the mere approach of a dominant individual causing anxiety-like emotion in the approachee. Heart rate changes following approaches by kin and by subordinate individuals were used as control measures. The second type of social interaction was allogrooming. Heart rate changes during grooming were compared to matched control periods. As expected, the approach by a dominant individual was sufficient to provoke a significant heart rate acceleration. The approach of the subject's kin or a subordinate nonrelative did not cause consistent heart rate responses. It was hypothesized that allogrooming has a tension-reduction function. In both subjects, heart rate deceleration was significantly more prominent while receiving grooming than in matched control periods.

1.2 Concepts related to emotion

Two concepts, motivation and stress, are closely related to emotion and should be mentioned briefly. Hunger, thirst, and pain, as described by Cannon, are motivational states, they can elicit a stress response, and are surely accompanied by emotions. Stress is defined by Averill, Opton, and Lazarus (1971) as a negatively toned emotional response. Indeed, all three terms, that is emotion, motivation, and stress, are only different aspects of the same phenomenon.

1.2.1 Motivation

According to Hamburg, Hamburg, and Barchas (1975), "emotion has several components: a subjective component, an action component, and a physiologic component appropriate to the action. The term emotion usually emphasizes the subjective component, but this is in fact the subjective aspect of a motivational pattern" (p. 237). Therefore, an emotion is an expression of a motivational state and this emotion helps to meet the adaptive tasks which are necessary for survival. A similar definition is given by Buck (1989): "emotion can be regarded as a process by which motivational potential built in to the organism is actualized when activated by a challenging stimulus. Emotion is thus a *readout* of motivational potential" (pp. 201–202). The author postulates a biologically based hierarchy of "primary motivational-emotional systems." These systems comprise reflexes, instincts or fixed action patterns, drives, affects, and effectance motivation.

1.2.2 Stress

We have already described the emergency reaction proposed by Cannon (1929) which is surely characteristic of a severe stress situation. This reaction is characterized by a general sympathetic discharge of the autonomic nervous system resulting in an increase of heart rate, rapid breathing, increased systolic blood pressure, vasodilatation in the skeletal muscle, and release of glucose from the liver. Many of these effects are at least caused partly by the discharge of epinephrine or adrenine (as called by Cannon) from the adrenal glands. According to Cannon, epinephrine "not only aids in bringing out sugar from the liver's store of glycogen, but also has a remarkable influence in quickly restoring to fatigued muscles, which have lost their original irritability, the same readiness for response which they had when fresh... (*This*) would give to the animal in which these mechanisms are most efficient the best possible conditions for putting forth supreme muscular efforts" (pp. 204–205). Especially relevant for our purpose is a footnote by Cannon in this context (p. 205): "If these results of emotion and pain are not "worked off" by action, it is conceivable that the excessive adrenin and sugar in the blood may have pathological effects."

During the late 1930s, Selye (1976) reported a nonspecific response in laboratory animals to different agents such as heat, cold, trauma, etc. This response which Selye called *stress* consisted in heightened activity of the anterior pituitary gland and the adrenal cortex with a heightened level of cortisol. The damaging agents eliciting the response were called *stressors*. Contrary to the definition by Selye, in engineering stress denotes all objective environmental factors acting upon the person without consideration of the resulting effects (Rohmert & Rutenfranz, 1975). Given a stress factor, the effects of stress, which will be individually different, are called strain.

The assessment of the stress factors is often possible with physical or technical measurements, whereas strain can only be assessed by physiological indicators and subjective ratings made by the individual. The following stress factors are important (Strasser, 1982): (1) Informational-mental, (2) social-emotional, (3) physical-situational (e.g., temperature), and (4) energetical factors (e.g., physical activity). The informational-mental and social-emotional factors represent psychological stress, whereas the physical-situational and energetical factors are classified as physical stress.

1.3 Work load: Theoretical background

According to the foregoing paragraph, there are four factors relevant in work resulting in four work load components: Total work load, physical work load, emotional work load, and mental work load. In contemporary workplaces the psychological components (emotional, mental) seem to be the most important. All components can be identified instantaneously by the joint on-line analysis of heart rate and physical activity.

1.3.1 Total work load

Heart rate is the parameter most often used to assess total work load in the laboratory and in the field. The electrocardiogram (ECG), which is used for the measurement of heart rate, is a very strong biological signal and, therefore, can be easily detected.

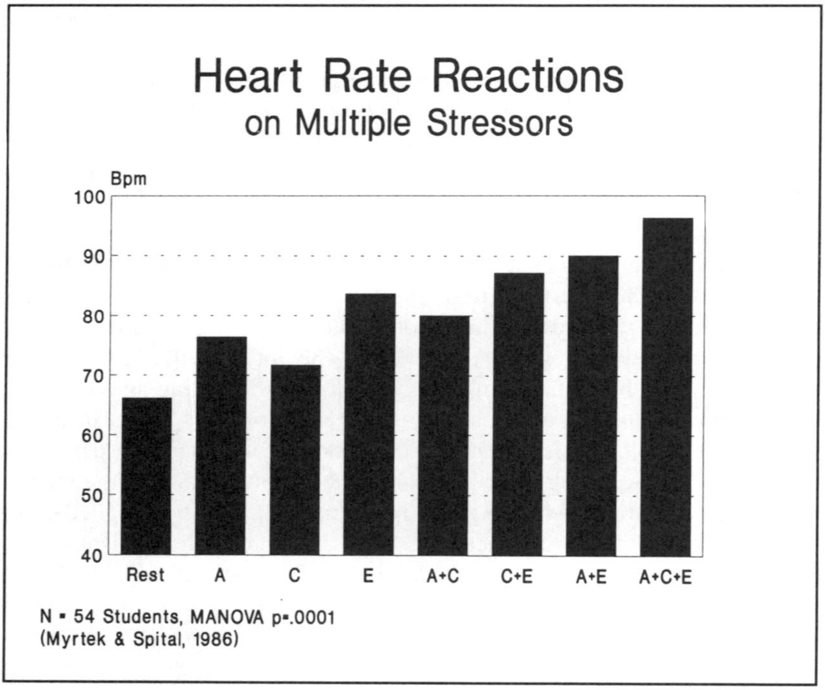

Figure 1. Heart rate reactions on multiple stressors: Mental arithmetic (A), cold pressor test (C), ergometric exercise with 25 watts (E), and combinations of all stressors. From Myrtek, Brügner, & Müller, 1996a. Reproduced with permission from *Ambulatory Assessment* by Fahrenberg & Myrtek, ISBN 0-88937-167-9, p. 116. Copyright 1996 by Hogrefe & Huber Publishers, Seattle, Toronto, Göttingen, Bern.

Several authors have demonstrated that heart rate reactivity in a stressor combination, for example, work on a bicycle ergometer (physical stress) and mental arithmetic (psychological stress), was higher than heart rate reactivity either in the ergometer or in the arithmetic condition (Bartenwerfer, 1963; Blix, Stromme, & Ursin, 1974; Roth, Bachtler, & Fillingim, 1990; Turner, Carroll, Hanson, & Sims, 1988). In an own laboratory study, we used the stressors mental arithmetic, cold pressor, and low grade ergometric exercise (Myrtek & Spital, 1986). Heart rate reactivity was significantly higher for all stressor combinations as compared to heart rate reactivity of the single stressors (see Figure 1). The combination of all three stressors yielded the highest heart rate reactivity which was significantly higher than each double stressor combination. Generally, heart rate reactivity elicited by a stressor combination was nearly an additive combination of the respective reactivity elicited by the single stressors. This experiment shows that heart rate reflects both psychological and physical work load.

1.3.2 Physical work load

Physiologically, there is a linear relation between physical work load and oxygen uptake (Mellerowicz, 1975). The latter is linearly related to cardiac output. On the other hand, cardiac output is widely dependent on heart rate. Therefore, heart rate is a measure of physical work load, when emotional or mental work load are absent. During psychological work load, heart rate increases above the level indicated by the oxygen uptake. This phenomenon is called *additional heart rate* (e.g., Turner et al., 1988). Compared to physical activity during which any increase in activity increases oxygen consumption in a monotone fashion, oxygen uptake during an increase in psychological work load is only slightly higher than without this increase (caused by an increase of muscle tone).

Figure 2 shows the relation between physical exercise on a bicycle ergometer and heart rate for three subjects. Subjects worked for six minutes with a load of 100 watt, two minutes with 150 watt, two minutes with 175 watt and so on, with an increase of 25 watt every two minutes (Myrtek & Nahrwold, 1974). Heart rate was taken in the last minute of each stage. As can be seen from the Figure, heart rate is indeed linearly correlated with physical work load. There are also differences in the physical capacity of the subjects. Subject #3 reveals a heart rate of 60.5 bpm at rest and of 174.0 bpm at 250 watt. For subject #1 the figures are 70.0 and 193.0 bpm, respectively. The lowest physical capacity shows subject #2 with a heart rate of 73.5 bpm at rest and 208.0 bpm at 250 watt.

We have already stated that heart rate reflects both psychological and physical work load. The greatest part of heart rate reactivity in a given situation, however, is due to the physical and not to the psychological work load component. During strenuous physical exercise, the amount of heart rate increase due to psychological work load is negligible compared to the amount due to physical work load. The linear relationship between physical activity and oxygen uptake, whereby this uptake is hardly influenced by psychological work load components, enables the estimation of the true physical work load by the measurement of oxygen uptake. This method is called indirect calorimetry.

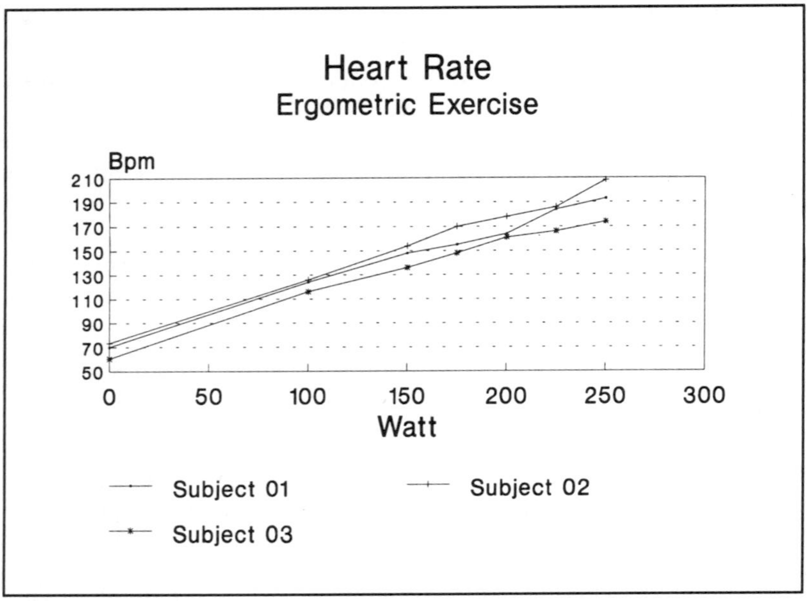

Figure 2. Heart rate (beats/min) and physical activity (watt) during ergometric exercise on a bicycle ergometer for three male students.

Under field conditions, however, measurements of oxygen uptake are difficult to obtain because subjects are forced to wear a mask. Therefore, several authors tried to assess physical work load by the subjects' physical activity. Avons, Garthwaite, Davies, Murgatroyd, and James (1988) demonstrated that physical activity assessed with very simple actometers already showed significant correlations with oxygen uptake. LaPorte and coworkers (1979, 1982; LaPorte, Montoye, & Caspersen, 1985) used relative simple motion detectors capable of detecting motion but not the intensity of motion. Using several samples, significant correlations between physical activity and energy expenditure were demonstrated. These methods are somewhat simple but with the use of more sophisticated measurement concepts it is possible to strongly enhance the correlation between physical activity and energy expenditure. With the use of accelerative sensors, very high correlations between oxygen uptake and physical activity were observed under laboratory conditions using treadmill ergometry (Tryon, 1991).

1.3.3 Emotional work load

The essence of this book deals with the measurement of the emotional work load component in everyday life. This assessment is more complicated than the measurement of the other components. A special monitoring device, the *Freiburg Monitoring System* (FMS; Myrtek et al., 2001) was developed by the Psychophysiological Research Group in Freiburg. As already mentioned in the Preface, the method is based on the simultaneous on-line comparison of heart rate and physical activity in order to assess heart rate increases which are not caused by physical activity, i.e., the *additional heart rate* (AHR). The on-line algorithms used for AHR are described in detail in Chapter 3 (Methods).

1.3.4 Mental work load

Many authors claim that a decrease in heart rate variability is an indicator of mental work load (Meshkati, 1988; Strasser, 1982; Wilson, 1988). We have shown in the above cited laboratory study (Myrtek & Spital, 1985) that the decrease of heart rate variability (operationalized by the mean squared successive differences, MSSD) during mental arithmetic was higher than during a cold pressor test. Attenuation of the T-wave amplitude of the ECG is also claimed to be an indicator of mental work load. However, our extensive studies with many different samples have shown that T-wave amplitude is not a valid indicator (Myrtek, Brügner, & Müller, 1996b). The question whether our emotional work load component will perhaps embrace the mental work load component, too, will be discussed later on.

1.4 Summary

The first chapter deals with definitions and models relevant for this book. There is as yet no satisfactory definition of what an emotion might be. Emotion research has to deal with several problems such as emotion induction, the interaction of the response systems (verbal-cognitive, physiological, behavioral), and the question of different physiological responses for different emotions. An important aspect is that emotional reactions in everyday life rely on self-reported emotional events. This implies that subjects can only report emotions they are aware of. It has been shown, however, that emotion perception is not always linked to physiological changes but seems to be essentially a function of cognitive schemas.

From an evolutionary point of view emotions have a protective function. Emotions mobilize disparate response systems to events that pose a threat to survival. Results show that emotional tachycardia is present in reptiles, birds, and mammals but not in amphibians and fish. The facial expression of emotions are obviously inborn and serve emotional communication.

Closely related to emotion are the concepts of motivation and stress. These terms seem to only refer to different aspects of the same phenomenon. Some authors claim that an emotion is an expression of a motivational state in which the emotion helps to activate adaptive tasks necessary for survival. The emergency reaction described by Cannon is a strong stress situation but represents a way of coping with a threatening situation. Whereas Cannon points to the sympathetic autonomic nervous system and the discharge of epinephrine, Selye focused on the anterior pituitary gland and the adrenal cortex. According to Selye, stress means a nonspecific response of the organism elicited by a stressor. In engineering, however, stress denotes the objective environmental factors acting upon the person. Stress elicits organismic responses which are called strain. We prefer this latter definition.

In the present book, a break down of the different work load components will be given. Heart rate is at the same time a sensitive parameter of both physical (energetical) and psychological (emotional, mental) work load and by this represents an indicator of total work load. In the absence of a psychological work load component, physical work load is linearly related to heart rate and oxygen consumption. However, if psychological work load is also present during physical work load, heart rate increases above the level indicated by the oxygen uptake resulting in the so-called *additional heart rate* (AHR). It has been shown that physical activity measured with a system of accelerative sensors is highly correlated with oxygen uptake. Therefore, physical activity represents the physical or energetical work load component. Many authors have claimed that a decrease of heart rate variability might be an indicator of mental work load. Whether there is truth in this will be discussed in Chapter 3.

Chapter 2

Basic physiological principles

2.1 Nervous control of the heart

Heart activity is regulated by both the sympathetic and parasympathetic division of the autonomic nervous system (ANS). Under normal conditions both divisions exhibit tonic activity, whereby the parasympathetic supply is inhibitory in its action and the sympathetic supply is stimulatory.

2.1.1 Parasympathetic fibers (nervus vagus)

The preganglionic fibers arise from the vagal motor nuclei and the nucleus ambiguus (nA) in the medulla oblongata and pass via the vagus to the cardiac ganglia. After transmission across the synapses, postganglionic fibers go out to the cells in the sinoatrial and atrioventicular nodes. Within the ventricular muscle no vagal fibers have been found.

Stimulation of the vagus (electrically or by the administration of acetylcholine) results in a decrease of heart rate, a diminution in the strength of the atrial contraction, and in a reduction in the conduction velocity through the AV node. Vagus nerve stimulation suppresses the development of the pacemaker potential in the sinus node through an increase of the permeability of the cell membrane to potassium ions (Antoni, 1997; Marshall, 1968).

Vagal tone of the heart derives from ongoing activity in peripheral sensory receptors (arterial baroreceptors, arterial chemoreceptors) and from other groups of central neurons. Stimulation of the arterial baroreceptors by rises in arterial blood pressure increases cardiac vagal outflow. Denervation of the baroreceptor reduces but does not abolish cardiac vagal discharge. Hypocapnia produced by hyperventilation causes tachycardia and reduction in cardiac vagal efferent activity. Vagal tone is also reduced by anesthetics presumably by reduction of tonic influences from other parts of the nervous system. Decerebration produces a vagally mediated fall in heart rate. Lesions in the hypothalamus (hypothalamic defense area) also produce cardiac slowing, whereas stimulation in this area inhibits cardiac vagal activity (Taylor, Jordan, & Coote, 1999).

2.1.2 Sympathetic nerves

Preganglionic fibers originate from the lateral horn cells of the thoracic spinal cord. These fibers synapse in the lateral sympathetic chains and the postganglionic fibers run to the sinoatrial and atrioventricular nodes and bundle of His. Fibers accompanying the branches of the bundle of His innervate the ventricular muscle. The lateral horn neurons themselves are controlled by neurons from the ventral medulla oblongata.

Stimulation of the sympathetic nerves (electrically or by administration of epinephrine or norepinephrine) causes an opposite effect than stimulation of the vagus: heart rate, force of contraction, and conduction velocity through the AV node are increased. Sympathetic nerve stimulation causes an increased rate of membrane depolarization during diastole in the pacemaker cells (Antoni, 1997; Marshall, 1968). Stimulation of the right sympathetic nerves especially causes increased heart rate and augments atrial force of contraction. The left sympathetic cardiac nerves augment ventricular contractions and also increases conductance and rate via the AV node (Taylor et al., 1999).

2.1.3 Central control of the cardiovascular and respiratory systems

The effectiveness of respiratory gas exchange is determined by the rates and patterns of lung ventilation and blood perfusion. Therefore, respiratory and cardiac rhythms are related to guarantee an optimal oxygen uptake. The neural substrate for respiratory rhythm generation lies in the medulla oblongata. Afferent fibers transmitting sensory information arises from the heart (mechano- and chemoreceptors in the walls of the atria and ventricles), vascular, and ventilatory systems (mechano- and chemosensitive sensory afferents throughout the respiratory tract). These circulatory and respiratory afferents are located in the trigeminal, glossopharyngeal, and vagus nerves. The arterial baroreceptors are located in the walls of the carotid sinus and aortic arch. Arterial chemoreceptors are located in the carotid and aortic bodies. The cardiorespiratory afferents terminate in the brain stem, in the nucleus of the solitary tract (NTS), and in the trigeminal nucleus. Vagal afferents terminate predominantly in the caudal two-thirds of the NTS and glossopharyngeal afferents in the rostral two-thirds (Taylor et al., 1999).

Any acute rise in arterial pressure increases the baroreceptor discharge rate and this enhances the vagal output to the heart and inhibits the sympathetic outflow to the heart and the vasculature (baroreceptor reflex). The baroreflex is very rapid with a latency between baroreceptor stimulation and onset of vagal bradycardia of 0.5 s or less. The latency for changes in sympathetic vasomotor nerve activity is about 1.5 s. A fall in blood pressure causes baroreceptor unloading and reduces the baroreceptor input to the brain stem. This results in tachycardia due to reduced vagal inhibition and increased sympathetic activity. Myocardial contractility increases due to the sympathetic activity. Furthermore, in most laboratory animals the baroreflex elicits a sympathetically mediated vasoconstriction involving the skeletal muscle, skin, kidneys, and the splanchnic vasculature. By this peripheral resistance is raised (Levick, 1995).

The ventilatory and vascular control systems are centrally coupled. The modification of cardiovascular control by the respiratory system dominates but stimulation of cardiovascular afferents can also modify the respiratory system. Respiratory sinus arrhythmia is due to respiratory modulation of the vagal parasympathetic innervation of the heart. Cardiac vagal efferent fibers fire preferentially during expiration. During inspiration the membrane potential of the vagal preganglionic neurons in the medulla oblongata is hyperpolarized due to the arrival of acetylcholine-mediated inhibitory postsynaptic potentials possibly from the NTS. This makes the neurons less amenable to excitatory inputs during inspiration. The neurons are excited by stimulating the baroreceptors (through rises in blood pressure) or the arterial chemoreceptors (by hypoxia). Moreover, cardiac vagal efferent activity is inhibited by lung inflation (through afferents from lung stretch receptors) resulting in a tachycardia (Taylor et al., 1999).

In the hypothalamus there are at least two regions which are involved in cardiovascular regulation. The hypothalamic depressor area is located in the dorsal part of the anterior hypothalamus and receives input from the NTS. Stimulation of this area activates the cardiac vagal fibers and inhibits sympathetic outflow. Especially relevant is the hypothalamic "defense area" in the anterior perifornical region. Electrical stimulation of this area in a conscious cat evokes tachycardia, hypertension, vasodilatation in the skeletal muscle, and behavioral manifestations of fear or rage. This reaction is known as alarm or fear-fight-flight response as mentioned earlier. The defense area is probably activated by the amygdala of the limbic system (see part 2 of this Chapter). Stimulation of the defense area indirectly inhibits the neurons in the NTS that are excited by the input from the baroreceptors (Levick, 1995).

2.1.4 Afferent fibers in the ANS

The afferent fibers (visceral afferents) running in the autonomic nerve strands have their cell bodies in the sensory ganglia of the cranial and spinal nerves and belong to the somatic system. Most of the visceral afferents are mechanoreceptors measuring either the pressure (e.g., carotid sinus, urinary bladder) or the volume in hollow muscular organs (e.g., digestive system, right atrium, lung). Some afferents originate from chemical sensors, e.g., arterial chemoreceptors in the carotid and aortic bodies (Bard, 1968; Jänig, 1997).

2.1.5 Epinephrine and norepinephrine from the adrenal medulla

The secretory cells of the adrenal medulla are the morphologic homologues of the postganglionic sympathetic neurons and, therefore, receive preganglionic fibers directly from the splanchnic nerves. Epinephrine and norepinephrine act upon any effector in the same way as nerve impulses conducted by postganglionic adrenergic fibers. However, epinephrine has special effects which cannot be produced by impulses in postganglionic sympathetic neurons. Heart rate and force of contraction of the heart are increased, blood flow through the skeletal muscles is enhanced by dilatation of the arteries, bronchioles are dilated, glycogenolysis in the liver and the skeletal muscles is augmented, and lipolysis in the fatty tissue is enhanced. These effects are transmitted by ß-receptors. Norepinephrine only acts via α-receptors and causes constriction of the venes and arteries especially in the skin and in the digestive system (Bard, 1968; Jänig, 1997).

2.2 Neurophysiology of emotion

Unpleasant emotions are associated with a defensive system which is active in fear and anxiety. Behaviors such as withdrawal, defensive aggression, and escape from pain are dependent on this system. Pleasant emotions on the other hand are associated with an appetitive system and behaviors such as approach, nurturant behavior, and sexual activity (Lang, Davis, & Öhman, 2000).

It is assumed that the center of the defensive system is located in the amygdala, part of the temporal lobe. Sensory information from all modalities is received by the lateral and basolateral nuclei of the amygdala. These nuclei project to the central nucleus of the same structure. From the central nucleus projection goes to the hypothalamus and the brainstem. The specific signs of fear and anxiety are mediated by the latter. Electrical stimulation of the central nucleus of the amygdala causes tachycardia, blood pressure elevation, and pupil dilation (by the lateral hypothalamus); bradycardia and defecation (by the dorsal motor nucleus of vagus and the nucleus ambiguus); behavioral and EEG arousal (by the locus coeruleus, the lateral dorsal tegmental nucleus, and the basal forebrain); increased startle response (by the nucleus reticularis pontis caudalis); facial expression of fear (by the facial motor nucleus); and release of corticosteroids (by the nucleus paraventricularis of the hypothalamus). Lang and coworkers assume that fear (a reaction to an explicit threatening stimulus with short term activation) is related to the central nucleus of the amygdala. Anxiety (a more general state of distress with long term activation), however, is assumed to be related to the bed nucleus of the stria terminalis (part of the extended amygdala). This nucleus projects over the same brain structures as mentioned above for the central nucleus.

The defensive system is an old part of the brain and evolved to serve the needs of simpler organisms long before the primates gained enough neocortex to enable language or rational thought. In humans this fear circuitry can be activated not only by the appropriate sensory input but also by imaginal representations and language. An activation of the circuitry is also possible without the participation of the neocortex. According to LeDoux (cited after Lang et al., 2000) an activation of the fear circuitry in rodents by stimuli associated with nociceptive events (conditioned stimuli) is also possible despite severance of the connections between the circuitry and the sensory cortex. Obviously, the primitive sensory thalamus is sufficient to provide the necessary input to the amygdala. Therefore, fear responses might occur without the conscious recognition of the stimulus.

2.3 Summary

The sympathetic and parasympathetic (nervus vagus) division of the autonomic nervous system (ANS) both exhibit tonic activity on the heart. Stimulation of the vagus results in a decrease of heart rate. Moreover, strength of the atrial contraction and conduction velocity through the AV node is reduced. Stimulation of the sympathetic nerves has an opposite effect. Heart rate, force of contraction, and conduction velocity through the AV node are increased.

An acute rise in arterial pressure increases the baroreceptor discharge rate and this enhances the vagal output to the heart and inhibits the sympathetic outflow (baroreceptor reflex). This reflex is very rapid with a latency between receptor stimulation and onset of bradycardia of 0.5 s or less. A fall in blood pressure results in tachycardia through vagal inhibition and increased sympathetic activity.

The ventilatory and vascular control systems are centrally coupled. Respiratory sinus arrhythmia is due to respiratory modulation of the vagal innervation or the heart whereby vagal efferent fibers fire especially during expiration. In cardiovascular regulation the hypothalamic depressor and defense areas are involved. Stimulation of the depressor area activates cardiac vagal fibers and inhibits sympathetic outflow. Electrical stimulation of the defense area, however, evokes tachycardia, hypertension, and vasodilatation in the skeletal muscle. Laboratory animals also show manifestations of fear or rage during the stimulation (fear-fight-flight response). The system is activated by the amygdala of the limbic system.

The adrenal medulla producing epinephrine and norepinephrine is stimulated directly by fibers of the sympathetic splanchnic nerves. Both hormones act upon the effectors in the same way as nerve impulses conducted by postganglionic sympathetic fibers. The hormonal effects for epinephrine are transmitted by ß-receptors and for norepinephrine by α-receptors. Epinephrine has special effects: increase of heart rate and contraction of the heart, enhancement of blood flow through the skeletal muscle, dilatation of bronchioles, glycogenolysis in the liver, and lipolysis in the fatty tissues. Norepinephrine has no metabolic effects and only causes constriction of venes and arteries especially in the skin and digestive system.

Unpleasant emotions are associated with a defensive system located in the amygdala and pleasant emotions with an appetitive system. Projections go from the amygdala to the hypothalamus and the brainstem which mediate the specific signs of fear and anxiety. In humans this fear circuitry can be activated by an appropriate sensory input from all modalities or by imaginal representations, too.

Chapter 3

Methods

To begin with, the method will be outlined briefly. Heart rate is measured by an electrocardiogram (ECG) and motion detectors serve to measure physical activity. Both parameters are analyzed on-line by a portable mini-computer. The values for heart rate and physical activity for a given minute are compared with the values of the previous minutes. If the heart rate of a given minute exceeds the rate of the previous minutes without an accompanying increase of physical activity, an increase in heart rate due to emotional factors (*additional heart rate*, AHR) is assumed (Myrtek et al., 1988). In this case and under several other predefined conditions, a feedback signal (a beep) is sounded in order to prompt the subject to respond to several predefined questions, displayed on the screen of the device, concerning his or her subjective state and current behavior. This method allows physiological, psychological, and behavioral parameters to be monitored simultaneously.

3.1 Freiburg Monitoring System (FMS)

3.1.1 Apparatus

In most of our studies we used a small computer called Multi-Talent (MT, Zak Company, Simbach, F.R.G.). The MT was equipped with an LCD display (4 lines with 16 columns each), an analogue device which served for the on-line analysis of physical activity and heart rate (input channels for two ECG leads and physical activity), and a digital output channel for a time code. The first ECG lead was used for the assessment of heart rate, the second lead served for the measurement of the ST-segment amplitude. By means of a computer with interface, the MT was programmable with Z–80. Programs for the analysis of the physiological signals were stored in EPROMs; other memories served to store the mean values, standard deviations, and other parameters of each minute. The size of the MT was 9.0 x 17.0 x 2.7 cm with a weight of 600 g, batteries included. Additionally, in some of our studies, especially in those with patients, we used an Oxford Medilog 4–24 tape recorder to record the analogue ECG signals of two chest leads. These signals were used for the off-line analysis of arrhythmias. In order to synchronize data from the MT and the analogue ECG signals, a code signal was generated by the MT and stored on the tape recorder. The whole system was carried by the subjects in a leather bag.

Because the MT device has no longer been produced for some years, we have adapted the algorithms to the recorders VITAPORT–II (TEMEC Instruments B.V., Kerkrade, NL.; Becker Meditec, Karlsruhe, F.R.G.) and VARIOPORT (Becker

Meditec, Karlsruhe, F.R.G.). A description of these recorders is given by Stephan, Mutz, Feist, and Weiss (2001). Subjective state and current behavior of the subjects are now recorded with the hand-held computer Psion 3a, which is connected to the recorder. An additional development is that posture and motion are assessed by calibrated accelerometry (Foerster, 2001). A detailed description containing all information about hardware, algorithms, application of electrodes, examples for the recording of behavior and subjective state, primary and secondary data analyses, norm values, and so on is provided in the book *Freiburger Monitoring System* (FMS) (Myrtek et al., 2001).

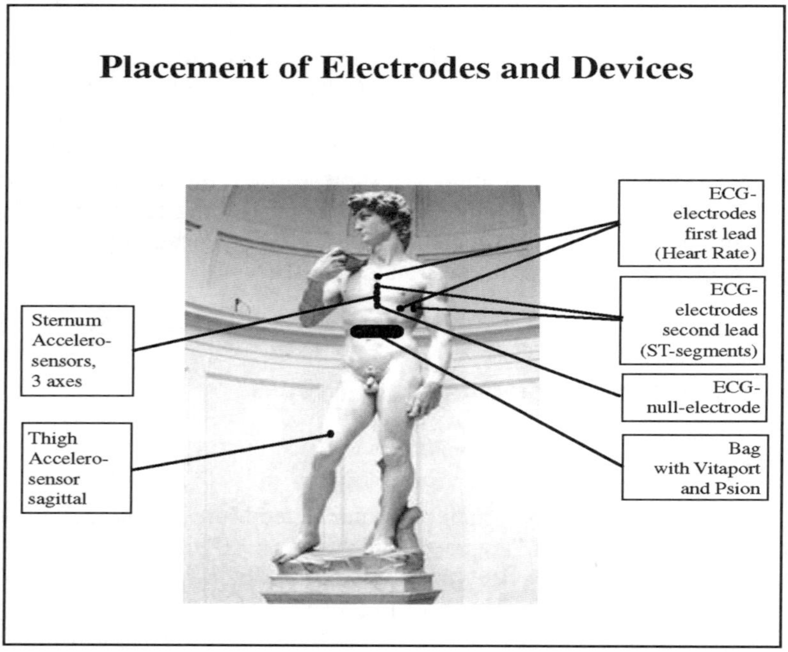

Figure 3. Placement of electrodes and sensors. From Myrtek et al., 2001. Reproduced with permission. Copyright 2001 by Peter Lang, Frankfurt/M.

3.1.2 ECG leads

ECG was recorded bipolarly with monitoring electrodes (Red Dot) attached on the chest of the subject. The first ECG lead was placed in a way to allow for a high R-wave amplitude (mostly V_4) in order to facilitate the recognition of heart rate during on-line analysis. The second lead was placed analogue to V_5. This lead served the analysis of the ST-segment amplitude. The negative electrodes for these leads are placed on the sternum beneath the fossa jugularis one below the other. Five electrodes, including a ground electrode (on the processus xiphoideus), were needed for each record (see Figure 3). It is important to test the quality of ECG lead attachment with an oscilloscope or when using VITAPORT–II or VARIOPORT with the VITAGRAF software. Furthermore, the ECG leads were tested in different body positions (supine, sitting, standing) to guarantee an optimal data quality for the analyses.

3.1.3 Physical activity

In our studies using the MT device, physical activity was measured by two motion detectors (accelerative sensors, Zak Company, Simbach, F.R.G.). The detectors were placed on the chest below the clavicle and on the thigh above the knee. Both detectors were coupled to give a common signal and were connected by wires to the analogue device of the MT. Each detector was sensitive to all three dimensions of space (three axes with piezo ceramic elements). The signal of the detectors was amplified and rectified in the analogue device. With the new devices, the placement of the detectors was changed to the sternum and the thigh in order to assess posture and motion (Foerster, 2001). For overall physical activity, the sensor output is combined on-line by vectorial addition.

3.1.4 On-line analysis of additional heart rate (AHR)

To understand the algorithms for AHR and for feedbacks, three requirements should be considered (Myrtek & Foerster, 2001):

1. Additional heart rate is an increase of the heart rate relative to the constitutional as well as the situational heart rate level. Therefore, the heart rate changes caused by physical activity due to metabolic demands have to be eliminated from the current heart rate.
2. The feedback signals prompting the subjects to rate their behavior should be continuously distributed throughout the day. Regular and nearly equidistant intervals between the feedback minutes would help to assess the behavior without gaps.
3. Besides feedback minutes initiated by AHRs (so-called *true feedbacks*), feedbacks without AHRs should be prompted (so-called *random feedbacks*).

On-line analysis of heart rate and physical activity was performed continuously by the MT device with a sampling rate of 256 Hz. The R waves of the first ECG lead were detected with the help of amplitude, slope, and curvature parameters which were continuously adapted to the changing shape of the QRS complex (moving average of 10 QRS complexes). Mean heart rate for each minute was computed from the number of R waves and stored. The impulses of the motion detectors were integrated for each minute and stored simultaneously.

For additional heart rate, the following parameters are relevant:

- Current heart rate of minute i:
- Heart rate level for minute i, defined as the moving average of the 3 minutes before the current minute: HRL_i

$$HRL_i = (HR_{i-1} + HR_{i-2} + HR_{i-3}) / 3 \qquad (1)$$

- Heart rate change of minute i: HRC_i

$$HRC_i = HR_i - HRL_i$$
$$= HR_i - (HR_{i-1} + HR_{i-2} + HR_{i-3}) / 3 \qquad (2)$$

- Physical activity of minute i: ACT_i
- Metabolic heart rate change caused by physical activity during minute i: HRM_i

$$HRM_i = ACT_i / CDIV_i \qquad (3)$$

- Parameter $CDIV_i$ is variable during on-line analysis according to rule 2 (see above; distribution of all feedbacks in the time domain) and rule 3 (see above; distribution of the number of *true feedbacks* in relation to the number of *random feedbacks*). This individual adaptation was reversed in the statistical analyses by setting CDIV to a fixed value of 30 in order to compare different subjects.
- Minimal heart rate change in minute i to classify this minute for a true feedback minute: $HRPLUS_i$:

$$HRPLUS_i = (90 + ACT_i) / CDIV_i$$
$$= HRM_i + 90/CDIV_i \qquad (4)$$

  with parameter $CDIV_i$ as mentioned above. Accordingly, in case of no physical activity, the minimal heart rate change is $90/CDIV_i$. Because $CDIV_i$ is limited to ≤ 30, the amount of HRPLUS is minimally 3 bpm.
- For additional heart rate of minute i (AHR_i), the amount corresponding to the factor, by which the current heart rate change (HRC_i) exceeds the minimal required heart rate change ($HRPLUS_i$) is calculated:

$$AHR_i = HRC_i / HRPLUS_i$$
$$= \{HR_i - (HR_{i-1} + HR_{i-2} + HR_{i-3}) / 3\}$$
$$/ \{(90+ACT_i) / CDIV_i\} \qquad (5)$$

  Note: In order to achieve integer numbers, AHR_i was multiplied by 10.
- For a minute with true feedback, current heart rate change (HRC_i) has to be higher than or equal to the minimal required heart rate change ($HRPLUS_i$):

$$HRC_i \geq HRPLUS_i \qquad (6)$$

  Or, in other words, current heart rate (HR_i) has to be greater than the minimal required heart rate change ($HRPLUS_i$) above the heart rate level for minute i (HRL_i):

$$HR_i \geq HRL_i + HRPLUS_i \qquad (6a)$$

  Or, with additional heart rate:

$$AHR_i \geq 1 \qquad (6b)$$

- Not regarded as true feedbacks are minutes with a strong increase in physical activity. It is required that current physical activity of minute i (ACT_i) is not higher than 10 units above the activity level (mean activity of the preceding 3 minutes):

$$ACT_i \leq (ACT_{i-1} + ACT_{i-2} + ACT_{i-3}) / 3 + 10 \qquad (7)$$

- Moreover, minutes fulfilling the requirements for a true feedback minute but following a minute with high physical activity and high heart rate are excluded. This means that the heart rate of a true feedback minute has to be higher than the heart rate of the preceding minute:

$$HR_i \quad > \quad HR_{i-1} \qquad (8)$$

- The continuous distribution of feedback signals throughout the day (rule 2) is controlled by parameter $CDIV_i$. Basically, 10–20 minutes after the last feedback a new feedback is required. If an insufficient number of minutes fulfills the criteria (6) – (8), the minimal requirement according to (6) is lowered. This means that the minimal required heart rate change will be reduced by augmenting parameter $CDIV_i$. For adaptation of parameter $CDIV_i$, the relation between the minutes already recorded and those minutes fulfilling criterion (6), that is, AHR ≥ 1, is considered:

$$\begin{array}{ll} \text{If} & N_{total} / N_{AHR\geq 1} < 5 \\ \text{then} & CDIV_i = CDIV_i - 1 \\ \text{If} & N_{total} / N_{AHR\geq 1} > 10 \\ \text{then} & CDIV_i = CDIV_i + 1 \end{array} \qquad (9)$$

  whereby $CDIV_i$ is limited to the interval [1, 30]. The starting point at the beginning of the recording is $CDIV_0 = 23$. If there is no minute fulfilling the criteria (6) – (8), that is, no *true feedback* possible in the prescribed interval of 10–20 minutes after the last feedback, then a feedback is nevertheless given in minute 20. These feedbacks are treated as *random feedbacks*.

- For reasons of comparison but also to avoid possible conditioning, *random feedbacks* are given with no indication of an emotional event after three *true feedbacks*. These *random feedbacks* are given randomly in the interval of 10–20 minutes after the last feedback. If in this minute for *random feedback* the criteria (6) – (8) are fulfilled (*true feedback*), then the next following minute is used for *random feedback*.

- If the relation between *true* and *random feedbacks* is smaller than 5:2, then no further *random feedbacks* are given with the exception that within the interval of 20 minutes no *true feedback* is possible. In this case a *random feedback* is given in minute 20.

The numerical values of additional heart rate for single minutes vary according to the algorithm between "0" and HRPLUS (formula 5) and are not, therefore, normally distributed. However, averaging the values over many minutes as done for such segments as daytime, night time, etc., yields a normal distribution. These algorithms were used in our studies and were developed empirically in several additional, small studies, whereby considerations of the amount of heart rate increases during emotional states played a significant role. Figure 4 shows an example o a 23h record of a fifteen year old schoolboy.

3.1.5 Other ECG parameters

3.1.5.1 Heart rate variability (MSSD)

Mental work load is operationalized in our studies by the mean squared successive differences (MSSD). The difference between the instantaneous heart rates (bpm) over two successive RR intervals is computed and squared. These squares are summed up and divided by the number of the differences. Finally, the square root is formed:

$$\text{MSSD} = \sqrt{\{\Sigma_{i=2,\dots,n}(HR_i - HR_{i-1})^2 / (n-1)\}} \tag{10}$$

The dimension of the MSSD is beats per minute (bpm). We have not used the instantaneous heart rates in all of our studies, choosing instead to use the RR intervals directly (8.3 ms/min, caused by the off-line sampling rate of 120 Hz).

$$\text{MSSD}_{RR} = \sqrt{\{\Sigma_{i=2,\dots,n}(RR_i - RR_{i-1})^2 / (n-1)\}} \tag{10a}$$

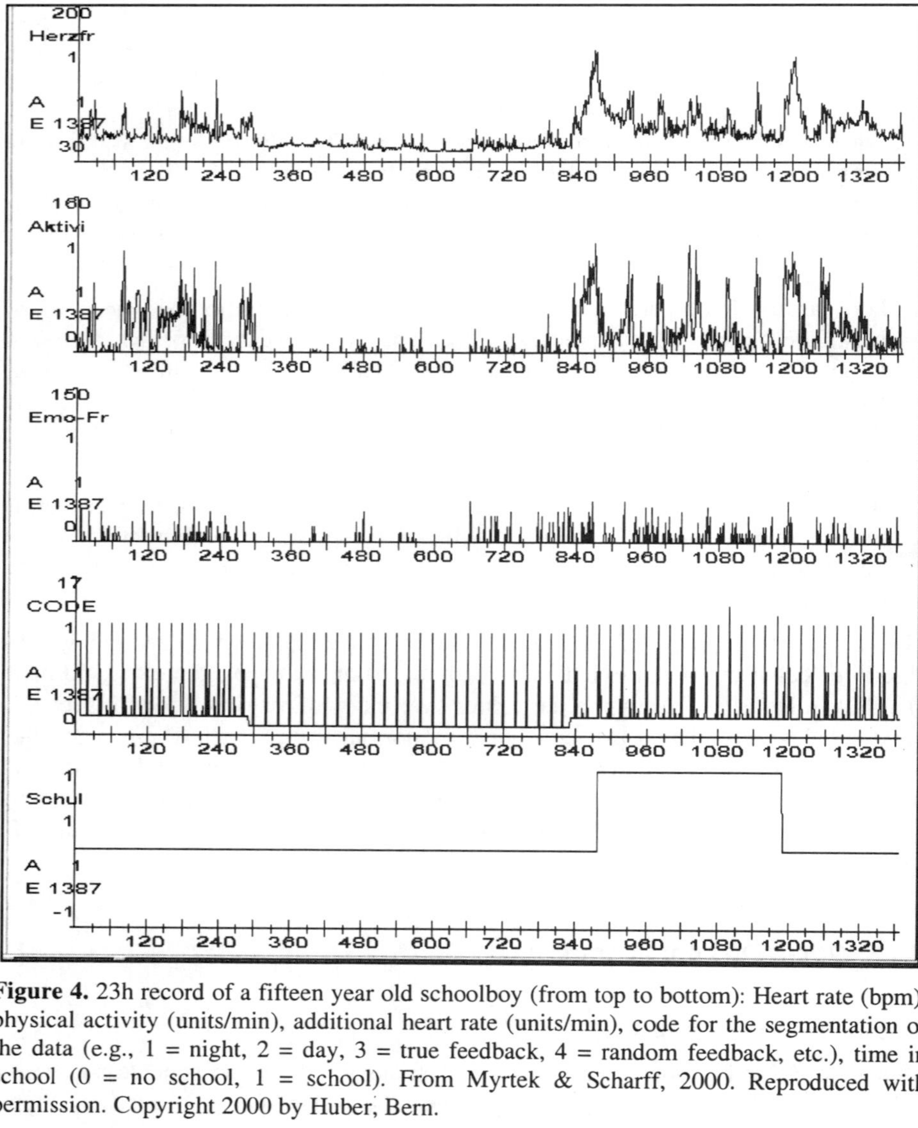

Figure 4. 23h record of a fifteen year old schoolboy (from top to bottom): Heart rate (bpm), physical activity (units/min), additional heart rate (units/min), code for the segmentation of the data (e.g., 1 = night, 2 = day, 3 = true feedback, 4 = random feedback, etc.), time in school (0 = no school, 1 = school). From Myrtek & Scharff, 2000. Reproduced with permission. Copyright 2000 by Huber, Bern.

3.1.5.2 P-wave amplitude

In several of our studies, the P-wave amplitude was shown to be a valid indicator of sympathetic activation (Myrtek et al., 1996b); this parameter might be valuable for field studies and stress-strain research. Naturally, P-wave amplitude is correlated with additional heart rate and physical activity because both parameters are associated with sympathetic activation. Therefore, an increase of the P-wave amplitude is an indicator of both emotional/mental and physical strain. A detailed description of the measurement is given by Myrtek et al. (2001).

3.1.5.3 ST-segment amplitude and ischemic episodes

In cardiology, depression of the ST-segment amplitude is an indicator of an insufficient blood supply to the heart (Deanfield et al., 1984; Gabbay et al., 1996). However, this interpretation begs caution. In our studies, we observed a significant depression of the ST-segment amplitude in some of our healthy 11-year-old schoolboys. This depression was also dependent on the body position. Similar results were reported by Csapo (1980) and Eggeling et al. (1988). It is interesting to note that women showed more ST-segment depression than men in our studies.

Only constant or descending ST-segment depressions are relevant in cardiology. Therefore, the normal slope of the ST segment of a subject is used for the interpretation of ST-segment depression. During on-line analysis of the ECG, ST-segment amplitudes of each heart cycle are measured 80, 100, 120, and 140 ms after the tip of the R wave. Reference points for the ST segment are measured 76 and 60 ms prior to the tip of the R wave. During off-line analysis the measurements of the ST segment are related to this so-called PQ knot, formed as the mean of the two points lying prior to the R wave. To serve as a reference, the two points forming the PQ knot should not show a difference greater than 0.035 mV. Otherwise, this heart cycle is omitted. For each minute of the record, the four ST-segment amplitudes of all heart cycles are averaged.

The difference is subsequently computed between the 140 ms point and the 80 ms point for each minute, whereby the amplitude of the 120 ms point should be > -0.5 mV and $< +0.7$ mV. These minutes are averaged and represent the normal ST-segment slope of the subject. The point of reference for ischemic ST-segment depressions is the ST-segment amplitude 100 ms after the R wave. Ischemic depression is postulated when the 100 ms point is ≤ -0.1 mV and the slope of the ST segment of this minute is not greater than the normal slope plus one *SD* of the slope. These minutes are marked in the record.

For clinical purposes, the determination of ischemic episodes is recommended. The first minute with an ischemic depression marks the beginning of an episode. The end of an ischemic episode is characterized by the minute which is followed by two minutes without ischemic depression. Single minutes in which there is no ischemic depression but which do occur within an episode do not interrupt the episode. Important parameters for ischemic episodes are the number of episodes, the minimal, mean, and maximal duration of the episodes as well as the minimal, mean, and maximal amplitude of the ST segment.

3.1.6 Assessment of behavior and subjective state

A feedback signal was emitted by the device every 10 to 20 minutes, resulting in an average of four feedback signals per hour requiring subjects' response. Subjects did not know that the feedback signals were triggered by their heart rate; they were only told that the signals served to monitor their daily activities. They had the possibility of canceling the feedback algorithm, for example, during the night. The average record had a length of 23 hours, whereby one additional hour was needed for attaching and detaching the device. On average there were eight hours of sleeping time, leaving 15 hours for feedbacks. With an average of four feedbacks per hour, maximally 60 feedbacks were obtained, resulting mostly in about 40 true and 20 random feedbacks.

The subject was requested by the acoustic feedback to describe his or her actual situation and subjective state. Questions were presented on the LCD-display of the device and were answered by moving a cursor and then pressing a key. Because there were four feedbacks per hour, questions had to be limited to a minimum and always had to be tailored to the respective subject samples. It took about 15 to 20 seconds to answer the questions, which were posed from the start of the monitoring till going to bed. Subjects were requested to start the feedback signals again upon awakening. By branching out the questions it was also possible to ask about more complicated issues.

Subjects were well instructed in the use of the device, and all questions together with the possible answers were demonstrated prior to ambulatory monitoring. In addition, a sheet of paper with the questions and the different answers was available. In the studies with patients, subjects were requested to activate the system by themselves if they perceived chest pain. These self-activations of the system were handled in the same way as were the true or random feedback signals, in which case the next feedback was given 10 to 20 minutes after the self-activation.

To give an impression of the questions posed, Figure 5 provides an example of a study with schoolboys (Myrtek et al., 1996a). In this study, we were especially interested in the TV consumption of the boys. At each signal, they were asked to provide the following information for the minute immediately prior to the beep: Feelings of excitement/arousal, enjoyment of the situation, physical activity, their whereabouts with subsequent questions tailored to the respective situation, and social circumstances. In the case of TV viewing, the boys were asked to disclose the TV station and type of program being broadcasted. All TV stations available in the town were listed on the screen of the device as were the different types of programs.

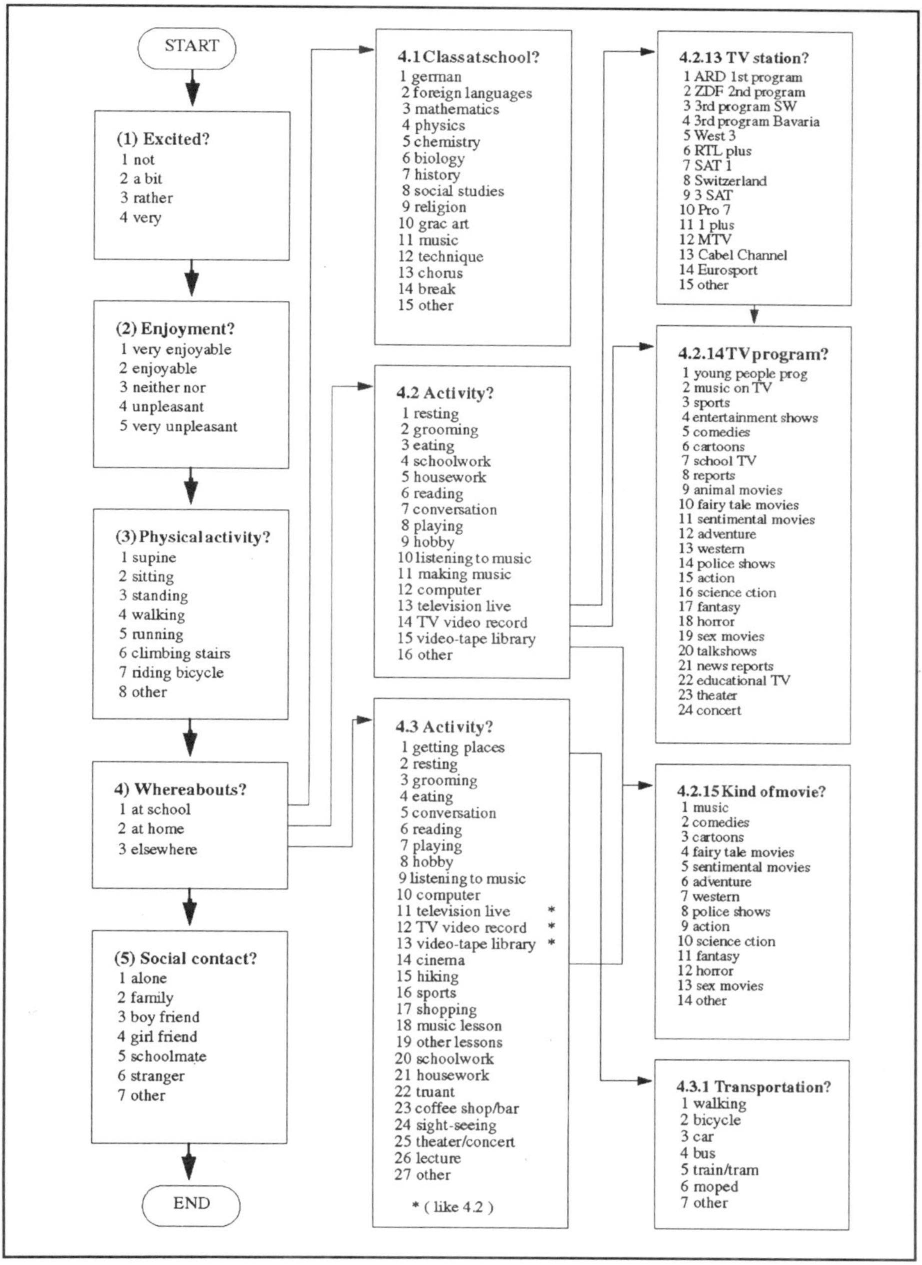

Figure 5. Example for the assessment of behavior and subjective state in schoolboys. From Myrtek et al., 1996a. Reproduced with permission from *Ambulatory Assessment* by Fahrenberg & Myrtek, ISBN 0-88937-167-9, p. 121. Copyright 1996 by Hogrefe & Huber Publishers, Seattle, Toronto, Göttingen, Bern.

3.1.7 Baseline

An important issue is the choice of a suitable baseline for the physiological changes during daily activities. An exactly measured and reproducible baseline is necessary because individual differences, say, in heart rate, are highly dependent on the actual physical condition of the subjects. Therefore, physiological parameters cannot be compared directly between different individuals and must be related to a baseline. In the literature ill-defined baselines are often used, for example, sitting for a short time at the workplace. In the present studies, the mean values of the physiological parameters assessed during deep sleep are used for baseline measurements, because heart rate at night generally reveals high stability coefficients. As demonstrated by Fahrenberg, Foerster, Schneider, Müller, and Myrtek (1985), the mean heart rate for an entire night revealed a stability coefficient of $r = 0.75$ in 42 students for an interval of one year. In another study with 27 cardiac patients, a stability coefficient of $r = 0.85$ for mean heart rate of the entire night was found for an interval of 11 days (Myrtek, Brügner, Fichtler, & Müller, 1994).

In the present studies, the hour of the night in which the heart rate mean reaches a minimum was assessed for each subject by means of a special computer program. The mean values of all physiological parameters for this hour, with exception of additional heart rate, were the baselines for the respective parameters assessed during daily activities. The variation of the baseline for heart rate defined in this way was high. In a sample of blue and white collar workers, heart rates varied between 42 and 80 bpm.

3.1.8 Data analysis

Artifact control of the physiological data was done with an interactive graphic program which shows all parameters of the 1387 minute record. Data which are thought to be artifacts were eliminated. To give an impression of the dropout and artifact rates, the rates of our study with industrial blue and white collar workers are cited (sample 17, see section 3.2).

Table 1. Missing data (MD) due to artifact control (mean of $N = 106$). From Myrtek et al., 1996a; modified. Reproduced with permission from *Ambulatory Assessment* by Fahrenberg & Myrtek, ISBN 0-88937-167-9, p. 122. Copyright 1996 by Hogrefe & Huber Publishers, Seattle, Toronto, Göttingen, Bern.

Parameter	*N* before	*N* after	% MD
Heart rate	146,166	142,790	2.31
Physical activity	146,166	142,790	2.31
AHR	146,166	142,790	2.31
MSSD	146,166	142,727	2.35
P–wave amplitude	146,166	141,046	3.50

Of 113 records, seven were total dropouts, that is 6.2% of the whole sample. Two dropouts were due to technical problems with wires and batteries, four dropouts due to problems with the electrodes, and one subject was not able to correctly answer the questions posed by the device. Table 1 shows the percentage of missing data after artifact control.

For behavioral categorization of the record, all variables of each feedback minute together with the variables of the previous and the following minute were assigned to a category according to the different behavioral information, for example, "daytime," "nighttime," "at work," "at home," etc. If the variables of two or more subsequent feedback minutes were classified in the same category, the variables of all minutes between the two feedback minutes were also assigned to that category. The variables assigned to each category were then averaged for each subject. Statistical analysis was done with these means and was carried out mostly using MANOVAs (general linear model analysis) in a two- or higher-factorial design (SAS Institute, 1993). Wilks' Lambda was used to determine the F values.

3.2 Samples monitored with the FMS

In the following the samples used in our studies will be shortly described. Besides the usual 23h monitoring, some special applications in the laboratory or at home are also mentioned.

3.2.1 Patients

(01) $N = 31$ cardiac patients (81% with myocardial infarction) monitored during their stay in a rehabilitation clinic for 23 hours; mean age 55.4 years ($SD = 6.1$).

(02) $N = 223$ cardiac patients (89% with myocardial infarction) monitored during their stay in a rehabilitation clinic for 23 hours; mean age 54.6 years ($SD = 6.9$). $N = 27$ of these patients were monitored twice.

(03) $N = 80$ patients with somatoform disorders monitored during their stay in a rehabilitation clinic for 23 hours; mean age 41.9 years ($SD = 9.1$).

(04) $N = 89$ patients with rheumatic diseases monitored during their stay in a rehabilitation clinic for 23 hours; mean age 49.4 years ($SD = 7.8$).

3.2.2 Healthy subjects

(05) $N = 36$ preschool boys ($n = 18$) and girls ($n = 18$); mean age 6.3 years ($SD = 0.1$). The children were monitored in their home environment during the presentation of selected films. Monitoring lasted 1.5 hours.

(06) $N = 100$ schoolboys in the 5th and 6th grades; mean age 11.1 years ($SD = 0.7$). 23h monitoring was done during a normal schoolday.

(07) $N = 100$ schoolboys in the 9th and 10th grades; mean age 15.4 years ($SD = 0.9$). 23h monitoring was done during a normal schoolday.
(08) $N = 50$ female university students; mean age 23.4 years ($SD = 2.7$). 23h monitoring was done at the university and during leisure time.
(09) $N = 96$ male university students; mean age 24.5 years ($SD = 2.2$). 23h monitoring started in the laboratory where students saw three films.
(10) $N = 120$ male university students; mean age 23.5 years ($SD = 2.4$). Monitoring was conducted in the laboratory during a discussion of relevant themes, e.g., unemployment in triplets and during the presentation of a film. Time base was reduced in this study from 60 s to 4 s. Monitoring lasted one hour.
(11) $N = 50$ male university students; mean age 23.7 years ($SD = 2.3$). 23h monitoring was done at the university and during leisure time.
(12) $N = 50$ female university students; mean age 22.3 years ($SD = 1.8$). 23h monitoring was done at the university and during leisure time.
(13) $N = 50$ male university students; mean age 23.3 years ($SD = 2.0$). 23h monitoring started in the laboratory where students saw a film.
(14) $N = 40$ male university students; mean age 24.7 years ($SD = 2.7$). 23h monitoring was done at an amusement park and during leisure time.
(15) $N = 60$ men and women (married couples); mean age 40.0 years ($SD = 11.5$). Monitoring was conducted in the home environment during the discussion of a relevant theme in their partnership and during the presentation of a film. Time base was reduced in this study from 60 s to 4 s. Monitoring lasted 1.5 hours.
(16) $N = 49$ train drivers, railway dispatchers, and bus drivers; mean age 46.6 years ($SD = 8.4$). 23h monitoring was done during work and leisure time.
(17) $N = 106$ blue and white collar workers from an industrial plant; mean age 50.6 years ($SD = 6.5$). 23h monitoring was conducted during work and leisure time.

3.3 Reliability of the FMS

3.3.1 Short-term reliability

23h monitoring of ECG and physical activity was carried out with N = 31 cardiac patients (mean age 55.4 years; sample 01) during their stay in a rehabilitation clinic. Most were admitted for myocardial infarction (Myrtek, 1990). Ambulatory monitoring began for all patients at about the same time of day. It was thus possible to analyze the synchronized time series of all patients for 22 hours from 2 p.m. until noon of the following day. For this reason, minute values were averaged for each of 5 minutes yielding a series of 264 5-minute values for each patient. Reliabilities were derived from Pearson correlations. Different time lags between the respective 5-minute periods were used to describe the reliability: 5 minutes, 1, 3, 12, and 22 hours.

The reliability coefficients generally are high with the exception of physical activity which shows great fluctuations from one minute to the next as well as heart rate variability. Heart rate variability measures are influenced by arrhythmias as shown by several patients, although beats with ventricular arrhythmias were omitted from the analysis. As may be expected, coefficients become smaller with increasing time lag. However, for many parameters a substantial increase of the coefficients from the 12 hour lag to the 22 hour lag is observed due to the change from day to night and vice versa.

Table 2. Short-term reliabilities for repeated measurements after five minutes till 22 hours. Correlation coefficients between the 5-minute periods are shown at the following times: (1) 2.00 p.m., (2) 2.05 p.m., (3) 3.00 p.m., (4) 5.00 p.m., (5) 02.00 a.m., and (6) 12.00 a.m. From Myrtek, 1990; modified. Reproduced with permission. Copyright 1990 by Elsevier, Oxford.

Parameter	Dimension	1 – 2	1 – 3	1 – 4	1 – 5	1 – 6
Heart rate	bpm	.94	.73	.68	.56	.63
MSSD	bpm	.48	.53	.53	.62	.36
ST-segment amplitude	microV	.97	.93	.83	.73	.81
P-wave amplitude	% R wave	.95	.87	.74	.20	.85
Physical activity	units/min	.67	.41	.26	–.02	–.41

The measurement points listed in Table 2 are daytime measurements with the exception of point 5 (time lag 12 hours) at which the measurements were made at night (2 a.m.). The smaller coefficient for heart rate might be due to individual differences in the reduction of the sympathetic tone or the increase in vagal tone at night. For heart rate, the coefficient for a repeated measurement after 5 five minutes is in the same range as observed in laboratory experiments. In a study with $N = 50$ male students a coefficient of $r = 0.94$ after eight minutes during rest was observed (Myrtek, 1975).

3.3.2 Long-term reliability (stability coefficients)

During their stay in a rehabilitation clinic, 27 male patients (mean age 53.8 years; sample 02) with ischemic heart disease underwent 23h monitoring of ECG and physical activity on two separate testing dates (Myrtek et al., 1994). Test-retest intervals ranged from 5 to 16 days for all but one patient whose test interval was 72 days. The overall mean interval was 11 days and the mean excluding the patient with the 72 day interval was 9 days. Test-retest stability was derived by Pearson correlations.

Table 3 displays the stability coefficients for daytime, nighttime and the total 23h mean values. The value for daytime heart rate, for example, is based on the average heart rate recorded in the 13 1/2 daytime hours. The coefficients for heart rate, heart rate variability (MSSD), ST-segment amplitude, P-wave amplitude, and additional heart rate are very high. These high coefficients are likely to be the consequence of a long recording time. The respective coefficients for nighttime data and the total recording time are similar. As could be expected, physical activity varied from day to day, resulting in low stability coefficients.

Table 3. Stability coefficients (repeated measurements after 11 days) for the total record (23 hours), daytime, and nighttime. From Myrtek et al., 1994; modified. Reproduced with permission. Copyright 1994 by Taylor & Francis, London (http://www.tandf.co.uk/).

Parameter	Dimension	23h	Day	Night
Heart rate	bpm	.86	.84	.85
MSSD	8.3 ms/min	.97	.98	.89
ST-segment amplitude	microV	.89	.88	.78
P-wave amplitude	% R wave	.90	.89	.86
Physical activity	units/min	.37	.46	.32
Additional heart rate	units/min	.79	.80	.75

Table 4. Stability coefficients (repeated measurements after 11 days) for physical activities: Lying (N = 21), sitting (N = 27), standing (N = 27), and walking (N = 25). From Myrtek et al., 1994; modified. Reproduced with permission. Copyright 1994 by Taylor & Francis, London (http://www.tandf.co.uk/).

Parameter	Dimension	Lying	Sitting	Stan-ding	Walking
Heart rate	bpm	.58	.83	.83	.59
MSSD	8.3 ms/min	.70	.98	.43	.65
ST-segment ampl	microV	.80	.89	.88	.95
P-wave amplitude	% R wave	.86	.87	.89	.83
Physical activity	units/min	–.06	.38	.32	.56

Table 5. Stability coefficients (repeated measurements after 11 days) for daily activities: Resting (N = 24), hygiene (N = 23), reading (N = 27), and eating (N = 27). From Myrtek et al., 1994; modified. Reproduced with permission. Copyright 1994 by Taylor & Francis, London (http://www.tandf.co.uk/).

Parameter	Dimension	Resting	Hygiene	Reading	Eating
Heart rate	bpm	.67	.73	.85	.76
MSSD	8.3 ms/min	.47	.16	.93	.93
ST-segment ampl	microV	.92	.86	.79	.89
P-wave amplitude	% R wave	.77	.79	.79	.80
Physical activity	units/min	.23	.10	.08	.34

An average of 49 true and random feedback signals were sent during daytime recording, meaning approximately one signal every 17 minutes. These feedbacks signals are the basis for our information on physical and daily activities. Some activities occurred only rarely and are thus omitted from our analysis. As can be seen from Table 4, stability of the ECG parameters during different physical activities is affected both by the number of minutes averaged for each activity category and by the type of activity. For example, the patients reported sitting for an average of about 26 minutes, whereas data related to the supine position is only based on an average of about four minutes. As can be seen, coefficients tend to be higher with more minutes averaged.

The data base for the coefficients in Tables 5 and 6 is generally small. The sample size is reduced for all activities but eating. Nevertheless, the data is worth examining. As already observed for physical activity, the ST-segment amplitude and P-wave amplitude are stable across the whole range of daily activities. The same is true for heart rate. The only exception is "taking a walk." As can be expected, physical activity shows low stability coefficients.

Table 6. Stability coefficients (repeated measurements after 11 days) for daily activities: Talking ($N = 24$), taking a walk ($N = 23$), working out ($N = 22$), and television viewing ($N = 15$). From Myrtek et al., 1994; modified. Reproduced with permission. Copyright 1994 by Taylor & Francis, London (http://www.tandf.co.uk/).

Parameter	Dimension	Talking	Taking a walk	Working out	Television
Heart rate	bpm	.73	.58	.73	.80
MSSD	8.3 ms/min	.94	.19	.01	.82
ST-segment ampl	microV	.90	.93	.72	.84
P-wave amplitude	% R wave	.75	.81	.75	.85
Physical activity	units/min	–.12	.52	.23	.71

Table 7. Stability coefficients (repeated measurements after 11 days) for different social situations: Alone ($N = 27$), together with other patients ($N = 27$), and together with other patients and staff ($N = 15$). From Myrtek et al., 1994; modified. Reproduced with permission. Copyright 1994 by Taylor & Francis, London (http://www.tandf.co.uk/).

Parameter	Dimension	Alone	Patients	Pat. and Staff
Heart rate	bpm	.81	.71	.75
MSSD	8.3 ms/min	.94	.95	.88
ST-segment ampl	microV	.86	.90	.94
P-wave amplitude	% R wave	.86	.86	.77
Physical activity	units/min	.39	.50	.17

The stability coefficients for being alone and being with other patients are high and in the same range as the total values for the entire daytime record (see Table 7). Due to the small data base of only 3 minutes, the coefficients for being with other patients and clinic staff together are smaller. For heart rate we can compare our ambulatory stability coefficients with various long-term stability coefficients measured in the laboratory (see Table 8).

Our stability coefficients measured at a mean test-retest interval of 11 days can be considered quite high. They are nearly in the same range as the short-term stability coefficients measured by the study cited above (Myrtek, 1990). Compared with the literature on long-term stability coefficients for heart rate derived from laboratory studies, our stability coefficients are still higher. This is most likely due to the broader data base in our study in which more minutes were averaged than usually done in laboratory studies. Several specific results deserve particular attention. The division into categories of physical and other daily activities indicates that some ECG parameters are highly stable in all situations, whereas others are dependent on the respective activity. Relative P-wave and ST-segment amplitudes are stable across all activities. Overall, the parameters derived from ambulatory monitoring can be said to have a good long-term stability. The coefficients are even higher than those observed in laboratory studies.

Table 8. Stability coefficients for heart rate from different laboratory studies.

Authors	Stressor	Interval	*N*	Stability
Hinz et al., 1992	Rest	3 months	26	.66
	Mental arithmetic	3 months	26	.76
Kamarck et al., 1992	Rest	1 week	18	.88
	Rest	2 weeks	42	.75
Kasprowics et al., 1990	Rest	4 weeks	48	.69
	Mental arithmetic	4 weeks	48	.72
	Rest	4 weeks	48	.62
	Mirror tracing	4 weeks	48	.71
	Rest	4 weeks	48	.60
	Bicycle exercise	4 weeks	48	.64
Mills et al., 1993	Rest	10 days	98	.68
	Standing	10 days	98	.55
	Rest	10 days	98	.68
	Mental arithmetic	10 days	98	.64
	Rest	10 days	98	.68
	Cold pressor	10 days	98	.53
Murphy et al., 1991	Rest	12 months	184	.41
	Video game	12 months	184	.75
	Rest	12 months	32	.45
	Video game	12 months	32	.65
	Rest	12 months	186	.41
	Video game	12 months	186	.55
	Rest	12 months	30	.40
	Video game	12 months	30	.63
Myrtek, 1985	Rest	1 week	48	.62
	Reaction time	1 week	48	.68
	Cold pressor	1 week	48	.79
	Number sequence	1 week	48	.78

3.4 Validity of the FMS

This section deals with the validation of the emotional, mental, and physical work load components. A first validation of the physiological parameters is given with the within-subject correlations of the parameters because certain expectancies concerning the amount of the correlations can be formulated. Generally, validation is only possible with help of external criteria. For this reason, states of physical, emotional, and mental strain must be induced in the subjects. If the parameters differentiate these different states, their validity can be assumed. The task of inducing different states is easy for the physical work load component. Much more difficulties emerge, however, with the induction of emotional or mental strain. Therefore, laboratory experiments designed to induce different emotional states were used for the validation of the emotional component. Moreover, certain categories of the field studies assumed to differ according to the emotional or mental component were used.

3.4.1 Within-subject correlations

Partitioning of covariance was used as summarized by Fahrenberg and Foerster (1982) and Stemmler and Fahrenberg (1989) for the within-subject correlations which give an account of the correspondence of the variables in the time domain, whereby covariation is pooled over all subjects and subject means are removed. These correlations are analogous to correlations derived by the *P* technique.

An important prerequisite for the assessment of the emotional work load component is the measurement of physical work load. Physical work load was assessed by physical activity measured with a system of accelerative sensors attached to the chest and the thigh. Because heart rate is determined primarily by physical work load, with lesser effects on heart rate caused by mental and emotional work load components, it must be postulated that a high correlation exists between heart rate and physical activity. Furthermore, the physiological parameters indicating either mental (mean squared successive differences of heart rate, MSSD) or emotional work load (AHR) should be independent of physical activity. Finally, the physiological parameters indicating emotional and mental work load should be unrelated, too.

The following results are based on eight different samples (see Section 3.2): White collar and blue collar workers (sample 17), railway employees (sample 16), 11-year-old schoolboys (sample 06), 15-year-old schoolboys (sample 07), two samples of male students (sample 11 and sample 09), and female students (sample 08).

Table 9 shows the within-subject correlations for eight different samples, the results being based on little over 23 hours. Actually, there was a high and reproduced correlation between heart rate and physical activity. Relatively low was the correlation for the railway employees. This is not surprising because the shaking of the locomotives or buses affects the accelerative sensors resulting in lower correlations between heart rate and physical activity. It must be mentioned that the high correlations were not caused through the joint analysis of daytime and nighttime values.

Separate analyses of daytime and nighttime values only showed very small differences for the correlation coefficients.

Table 9. Within-subject correlations for 1387 minutes, day and nighttime. From Myrtek et al., 1996b; modified. Reproduced with permission from *Ambulatory Assessment* by Fahrenberg & Myrtek, ISBN 0-88937-167-9, p. 291. Copyright 1996 by Hogrefe & Huber Publishers, Seattle, Toronto, Göttingen, Bern.

Samples	**Parameters**	*r*			
	Heart rate	**HR**			
50 White collar workers	Physical activity	.70			
40 Blue collar workers		.73			
49 Railway Employees		.69			
50 Boys 11 years		.81			
50 Boys 15 years		.77			
50 Students male		.74			
50 Students male		.74			
50 Students female		.77			
			PA		
50 White collar workers	Additional heart rate	14	.00		
40 Blue collar workers		14	–.02		
49 Railway Employees		14	.00		
50 Boys 11 years		13	.00		
50 Boys 15 years		14	.01		
50 Students male		15	.01		
50 Students male		15	.01		
50 Students female		16	.03		
				AHR	
50 White collar workers	Heart rate variability	–.27	–.15	–.03	
40 Blue collar workers		–.33	–.17	–.03	
49 Railway Employees		–.25	–.11	–.02	
50 Boys 11 years		–.28	–.19	–.05	
50 Boys 15 years		–.34	–.20	–.03	
50 Students male		–.60	–.36	–.07	
50 Students male		–.54	–.29	–.06	
50 Students female		–.62	–.41	–.10	
					MSSD
50 White collar workers	P-wave amplitude	69	.52	.07	–.14
40 Blue collar workers		73	.55	.07	–.22
49 Railway Employees		67	.53	.09	–.10
50 Boys 11 years		61	.52	.10	–.13
50 Boys 15 years		70	.57	.11	–.17
50 Students male		72	.58	.08	–.35
50 Students male		74	.62	.08	–.29
50 Students female		69	.55	.11	–.34

A consistent but small and expected correlation of about $r = 0.14$ was seen between heart rate and AHR. The correlation between physical activity and AHR, however, was zero. A small and negative correlation of about $r = -0.05$ existed between AHR and heart rate variability (MSSD). AHR and P-wave amplitude were correlated with about $r = 0.09$. The results show that AHR is a component which is neither related to physical activity nor to heart rate variability, thus confirming the above formulated expectations.

MSSD, however, was correlated negatively to a substantial degree with heart rate and physical activity. The correlation with physical activity especially affects the interpretation that MSSD is an indicator of mental work load because it cannot be assumed that higher physical activity will lead automatically to higher mental work load. The substantial positive correlations between P-wave amplitude, on the one hand, and heart rate and physical activity, on the other, as well as the small negative correlations between P-wave amplitude and MSSD do not affect the interpretation that P-wave amplitude is an indicator of sympathetic activation.

3.4.2 Induction of emotional arousal in laboratory experiments

3.4.2.1 Funny and erotic movies

Two laboratory experiments were conducted with $N = 48$ male students each (mean age 24.3 and 24.6 years; sample 09). Subjects watched three movies (30 minutes) in permutated order: A funny movie ("Some like it hot"), an erotic movie, and an emotionally neutral movie (landscapes of the Vosges mountains).

Table 10. Mean comparisons funny vs. erotic movie. From Myrtek et al., 1996b; modified. Reproduced with permission from *Ambulatory Assessment* by Fahrenberg & Myrtek, ISBN 0-88937-167-9, p. 292. Copyright 1996 by Hogrefe & Huber Publishers, Seattle, Toronto, Göttingen, Bern.

Parameters	Dimension	Condition	Funny	Erotic	p
Heart rate	bpm	Rest	64.85	67.24	.006
		Ergometer	71.77	75.91	.000
Physical activity	units/min	Rest	3.46	1.52	.004
		Ergometer	50.01	52.14	.011
AHR	units/min	Rest	2.63	3.14	.034
		Ergometer	0.92	1.33	.039
MSSD	8.3 ms/min	Rest	8.09	6.71	.000
		Ergometer	5.83	5.67	.530
P wave	microV	Rest	111.14	113.07	.606
		Ergometer	127.28	139.15	.006

The experiments were conducted under two conditions. The first sample watched the movies, sitting in a comfortable chair. The second sample continuously worked in the supine position on a bicycle ergometer with two minutes no load, two minutes minimal load of 10 watts, two minutes no load, etc. It was the intention of the second condition to show that AHR can be assessed under physical activity as well. Table 10 shows the mean comparisons between the funny and the erotic movie.

3.4.2.2 *"The silence of the lambs"*

In a study with $N = 50$ male students (mean age 23.3 years; sample 13), subjects saw at the beginning of the 23h monitoring a 60 minute section of the movie "The silence of the lambs" by Jonathan Demme with Jodie Forster as FBI-agent Starling and Anthony Hopkins as Dr. Hannibal Lecter (Zanda, 1999).

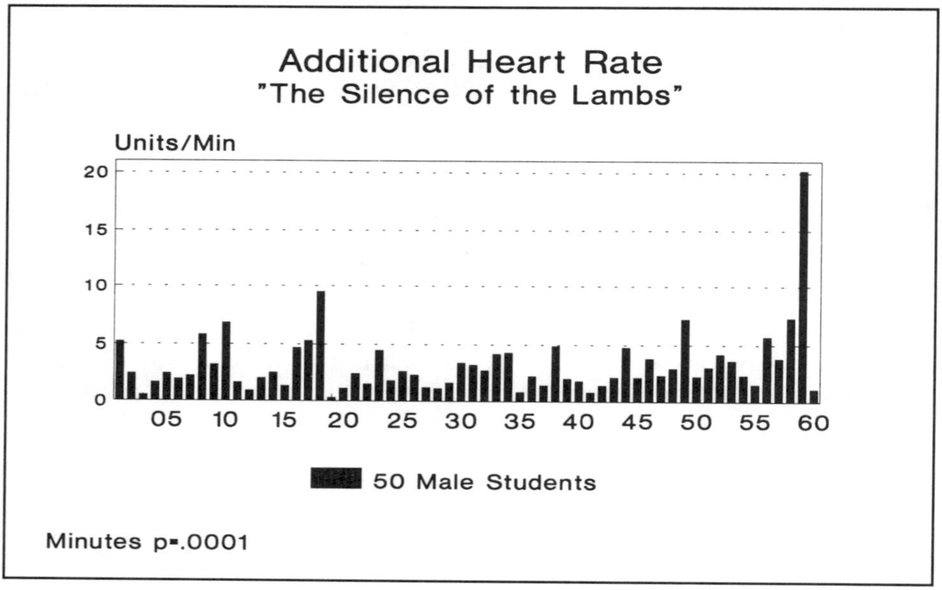

Figure 6. Additional heart rate during a 60 minute section of "The silence of the lambs."

As can be seen from Figure 6, striking differences exist between the minutes with some prominent spikes:

- Minutes 08–10: Starling finds a human head in an obscure storehouse in Baltimore.
- Minutes 16–18: Assault upon a woman by Buffalo Bill in Memphis.
- Minutes 33–34: Buffalo Bill torments a young girl imprisoned in a drawwell of his house.
- Minute 49: Starling meets Hannibal Lecter who is imprisoned in a cage.
- Minutes 58–59: Assault of Hannibal Lecter upon two guards who bring him his meal.

These minutes are especially exciting and further validate the AHR.

After viewing the film, subjects were requested to fill in a short questionnaire for evaluation of the film. Table 11 depicts the mean values and the correlations between these items and AHR. The film was rated predominantly suspenseful and rather exciting, disgusting, and frightening. AHR was higher in subjects who rated the film as more frightening and more suspenseful.

Table 11. Means of the evaluation items for "The silence of the lambs" and correlations between these items and AHR during the film ($N = 49$).

Evaluation of the film	Scale	Mean	*r*
Exciting	1–5, 5=absolutely	2.63	0.18
Frightening	1–5, 5=absolutely	2.47	**0.34**
Disgusting	1–5, 5=absolutely	2.59	–0.04
Enraging	1–5, 5=absolutely	1.29	–0.10
Unpleasant	1–5, 5=absolutely	1.55	0.16
Suspenseful	1–5, 5=absolutely	3.94	**0.32**

3.4.3 Testing hypotheses of expected differences between segments

According to the different observation categories assessed during monitoring, e.g., daytime, nighttime, working time, leisure time, categories of different physical activities, etc., mean values were computed for each category and each subject. These mean values of the different categories were compared using *t* tests for dependent samples and MANOVAs. The complete tables are given in Myrtek et al. (1996b). In the present section only the results of our meta-analyses are reported.

Effect sizes *r* were computed from the *p* values of the mean comparisons. Meta-analyses were conducted by means of a special program designed by Schwarzer (1989). The variance of the population effect size *R* was calculated according to the Schmidt-Hunter method. In the text, the following parameters are mentioned:

- Total *N* of all samples (*N*).
- Number of combined effect sizes (*K*).
- Population effect size (*R*) as the weighted average of all correlation coefficients: $\Sigma N_i r_i / \Sigma N$ (r_i = correlation coefficient of sample *i*). According to Cohen (1977), a population effect size of $R = 0.10$ is considered small, $R = 0.30$ moderate, and $R = 0.50$ high.
- Overall *z*-score of the standard normal deviation (*z*): $z = R * \sqrt{N}$.
- Significance of this *z*-score (one-tailed *p*).
- The mean standardized difference (*d*).

3.4.3.1 Daytime versus nighttime

A natural variation in sympathetic activity as well as in the degree of physical and presumably mental work load is given by the day-night cycle. Therefore, substantial differences in heart rate, physical activity, MSSD, and P-wave amplitude should be observed. For AHR no explicit hypothesis can be formulated because the REM phases at night show heart rate increases which would be interpreted as AHR by this method. Mean comparisons were made between daytime and nighttime for the samples cited in section 3.4.1.

Table 12. Meta-analyses for mean comparisons daytime vs. nighttime. From Myrtek et al., 1996b; modified. Reproduced with permission from *Ambulatory Assessment* by Fahrenberg & Myrtek, ISBN 0-88937-167-9, p. 293. Copyright 1996 by Hogrefe & Huber Publishers, Seattle, Toronto, Göttingen, Bern.

Parameters	*N*	*K*	*R*	*z*	*p*	*d*
Heart rate	435	8	.442	9.70	.00000	0.99
Physical activity	435	8	.442	9.70	.00000	0.99
MSSD	435	8	.373	8.05	.00000	0.80
P wave	435	8	.442	9.70	.00000	0.99

As can be seen from Table 12, the hypotheses were substantiated impressively for heart rate, physical activity, and P-wave amplitude. The meta-analysis revealed a weighted population effect size of $r = 0.442$ or $d = 0.99$ (N = 435). This effect size is high, because *d* values of about 0.20 are considered to be small, values of about 0.50 as medium, and values of about 0.80 as high. Consistent, although not always significant, differences were observed for MSSD. Only small differences between daytime and nighttime were seen for AHR.

3.4.3.2 Sitting versus standing versus walking

Variations in body position or body movements are naturally occurring stress factors which should document themselves in different levels of energetical strain. Therefore, distinct differences in physical activity and heart rate should be expected. Because sympathetic activation rises with increasing physical stress, systematic differences for P-wave amplitude are postulated too. No systematic effects are expected for the other parameters.

Table 13. Meta-analyses for mean comparisons sitting vs. standing vs. walking. From Myrtek et al., 1996b; modified. Reproduced with permission from *Ambulatory Assessment* by Fahrenberg & Myrtek, ISBN 0-88937-167-9, p. 295. Copyright 1996 by Hogrefe & Huber Publishers, Seattle, Toronto, Göttingen, Bern.

Parameters	*N*	*K*	*R*	*z*	*p*	*d*
Heart rate	316	8	.519	9.91	.00000	1.21
Physical activity	316	8	.519	9.91	.00000	1.21
P wave	316	8	.519	9.91	.00000	1.21

Table 13 shows that the hypotheses for physical activity, heart rate, and P-wave amplitude were confirmed. All parameters revealed a distinct gradual variation with increasing values from sitting to walking. As expected, no systematic differences were seen for AHR. However, for MSSD, systematic variations were observed with decreasing values for increasing physical stress. Theoretically, an increasing mental load might be postulated, which surely would be problematic in the given context.

3.4.3.3 *Working time versus leisure time*

For these comparisons (samples 16 and 17) it is more difficult to formulate clear cut hypotheses, because the various work and leisure activities are rather different. Most likely, a decrease in the energetical and mental work load components should be expected during leisure time together with a decrease of sympathetic activation. Therefore, during leisure time, lower physical activity and heart rate, higher values for MSSD, and lower values for P-wave amplitude should be expected. No explicit hypothesis can be formulated for AHR.

As expected, heart rate and physical activity were lower during leisure time for the blue collar workers and railway employees. No differences were observed for the white collar workers, because this group was mostly sitting during working time as well as during leisure time (see Table 14). P-wave amplitude was lower in all samples during leisure time. MSSD indicating mental work load, showed the expected difference only for the blue collar workers. For AHR surprisingly consistent and significant differences were observed with higher values during leisure time in all samples.

Table 14. Meta-analyses for mean comparisons work vs. leisure time. From Myrtek et al., 1996b; modified. Reproduced with permission from *Ambulatory Assessment* by Fahrenberg & Myrtek, ISBN 0-88937-167-9, p. 296. Copyright 1996 by Hogrefe & Huber Publishers, Seattle, Toronto, Göttingen, Bern.

Parameters	*N*	*K*	*R*	*z*	*p*	*d*
Heart rate	139	3	.357	4.31	.00001	0.76
Physical activity	139	3	.300	3.59	.00017	0.63
MSSD	139	3	.041	0.48	.31386	0.08
P wave	139	3	.404	4.94	.00000	0.88

3.4.3.4 *Staying at school/university versus staying at home*

Similar to the comparisons between working time and leisure time, differences in sympathetic activation and especially for the mental work load component might be expected. Accordingly, staying at home should reveal lower values for P-wave amplitude and higher values for MSSD. No distinct hypotheses can be formulated for the other parameters.

In four out of five samples (samples 06, 07, 08, 09, 11) P-wave amplitude was significantly reduced during staying at home as compared to staying at school or at the university. MSSD revealed differences for the student samples as expected but was not significantly different for the schoolboys (see Table 15). Staying at school or at the university generally revealed higher heart rate and higher physical activity than staying at home. The emotional work load component (AHR) showed a tendency for higher values for the student samples during their stay at the university as compared to staying at home but this was not true for the schoolboys.

Table 15. Meta-analyses for mean comparisons school/university vs. at home. From Myrtek et al., 1996b; modified. Reproduced with permission from *Ambulatory Assessment* by Fahrenberg & Myrtek, ISBN 0-88937-167-9, p. 297. Copyright 1996 by Hogrefe & Huber Publishers, Seattle, Toronto, Göttingen, Bern.

Parameters	*N*	*K*	*R*	*z*	*p*	*d*
MSSD	260	5	.276	4.52	.00000	0.58
P wave	260	5	.400	6.71	.00000	0.87

3.4.3.5 Social contacts with peers versus social contacts with strangers

It can be presumed that the emotional and mental work load components evoked in social situations differ according to the degree of familiarity between the interacting persons. Therefore, it can be postulated that the parameters AHR, heart rate, and MSSD will show differences between the familiar social contact with peers and the contact with unknown persons.

Table 16. Meta-analyses for mean comparisons social contacts: peers vs. strangers. From Myrtek et al., 1996b; modified. Reproduced with permission from *Ambulatory Assessment* by Fahrenberg & Myrtek, ISBN 0-88937-167-9, p. 298. Copyright 1996 by Hogrefe & Huber Publishers, Seattle, Toronto, Göttingen, Bern.

Parameters	*N*	*K*	*R*	*z*	*p*	*d*
Heart rate	84	5	.447	4.26	.00001	1.00
AHR	84	5	.380	3.56	.00018	0.82
MSSD	84	5	.484	4.66	.00000	1.11

AHR was indeed higher during the social contact with strangers in all samples than social contact with peers (see Table 16). Unfortunately, contacts with strangers are rather rare events leading to strong reductions in the number of observations and, therefore, the level of significance was not always reached. Still more pronounced than AHR were the differences for MSSD. In line with the expectations, heart rate showed differences, too.

3.4.3.6 High versus low TV consumption

Due to the often highly emotional content, television programs frequently produce emotional arousal irrespective of wether news reports or TV movies are viewed. It can be presumed, however, that the amount of evoked emotional activation will depend on the amount of TV consumption with higher consumption showing reduced activation due to habituation. Therefore, the hypothesis was postulated that groups with either high or low TV consumption will show systematic differences for AHR and heart rate with higher values for the latter groups (samples 05, 06, 07, 09, 17).

As expected, AHR and heart rate were higher in all samples with low TV consumption, although, due to the sample sizes level of significance was not always reached (see Table 17). No systematic differences, however, were observed for the other parameters. The most pronounced difference between low and high TV consumption was seen in the sample of children with an effect size of $r = 0.446$ or $d = 0.98$.

Table 17. Meta-analyses for mean comparisons high vs. low TV consumption. From Myrtek et al., 1996b; modified. Reproduced with permission from *Ambulatory Assessment* by Fahrenberg & Myrtek, ISBN 0-88937-167-9, p. 299. Copyright 1996 by Hogrefe & Huber Publishers, Seattle, Toronto, Göttingen, Bern.

Parameters	***N***	***K***	***R***	***z***	***p***	***d***
Heart rate	274	5	.204	3.41	.00032	0.42
AHR	274	5	.269	4.52	.00000	0.56

3.5 Special aspects of AHR

3.5.1 Distribution

Because AHR is a new parameter, the distribution might be interesting. Figure 7 shows a box plot and the frequency of mean AHR during the day for $N = 200$ schoolboys (combined samples 06 and 07).

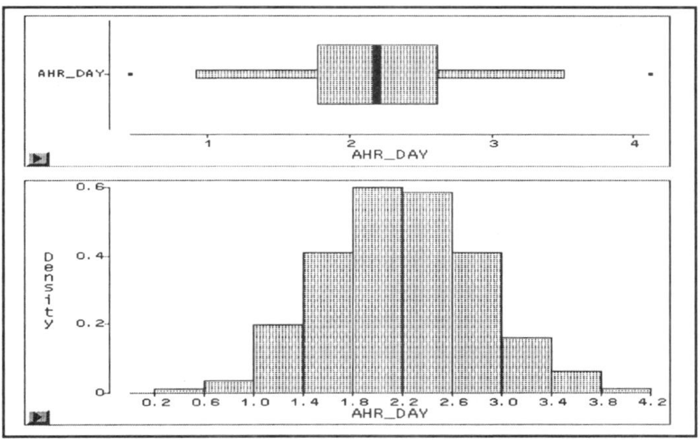

Moments			
N	200.0000	Sum Wgts	200.0000
Mean	2.2000	Sum	440.0089
Std Dev	0.6045	Variance	0.3655
Skewness	0.0745	Kurtosis	0.0036
USS	1040.7642	CSS	72.7250
CV	27.4779	Std Mean	0.0427

Figure 7. Distribution of mean AHR during the day for a sample of $N = 200$ schoolboys.

The statistical analysis reveals that AHR is normally distributed. For comparison, the distributions of heart rate and physical activity are also given (see Figures 8 and 9). Both parameters are normally distributed, too. However, the interindividual range of AHR is greater than the range of heart rate.

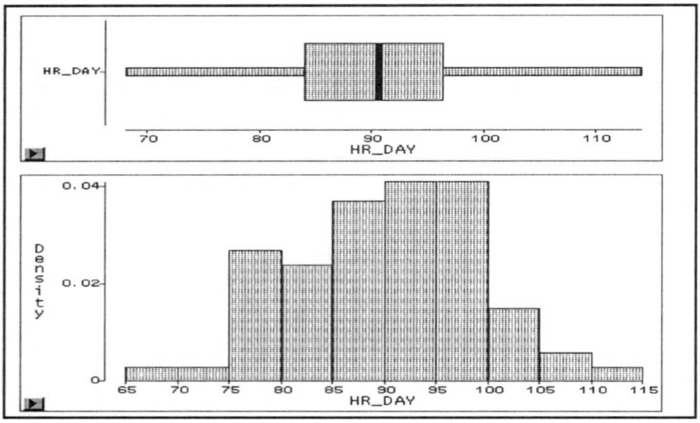

Moments			
N	200.0000	Sum Wgts	200.0000
Mean	90.2787	Sum	18055.7358
Std Dev	9.0137	Variance	81.2468
Skewness	0.0099	Kurtosis	-0.2995
USS	1646216.08	CSS	16168.1076
CV	9.9843	Std Mean	0.6374

Figure 8. Distribution of mean heart rate during the day for a sample of $N = 200$ schoolboys.

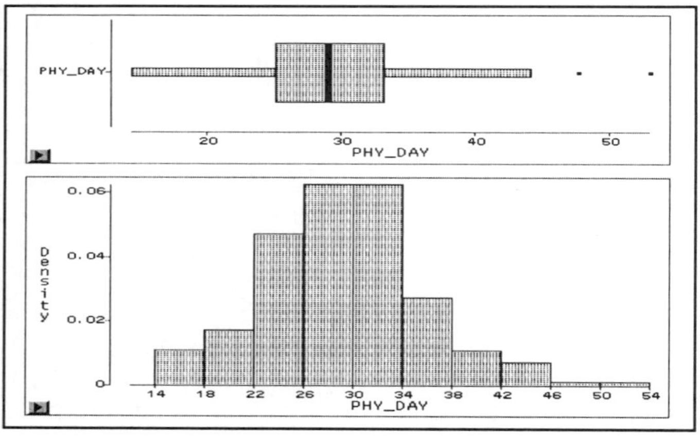

Moments			
N	200.0000	Sum Wgts	200.0000
Mean	29.4309	Sum	5886.1751
Std Dev	6.5254	Variance	42.5807
Skewness	0.3171	Kurtosis	0.6418
USS	181708.849	CSS	8473.5609
CV	22.1719	Std Mean	0.4614

Figure 9. Distribution of mean physical activity during the day for a sample of $N = 200$ schoolboys.

As stated in Chapter 3.1.4, AHR for a single minute varies between "0" and "HRPLUS" representing single emotional reactions. The interesting question might be posed as to how many of such reactions occur during the day (nighttime excluded). For the sample of 200 schoolboys, on the average 107 minutes with AHR were observed with a wide range from 26 to 185 events. In the following we will not consider single events but the averaged values for the different segments.

3.5.2 Age dependency of AHR

Emotional reactivity of the heart (AHR) is dependent on age. In the next Figures, the following age groups are considered:

- 11-year-old schoolboys $N = 100$ (sample 06),
- 15-year-old schoolboys $N = 100$ (sample 07),
- 24-year-old students, $N = 100$ (combined samples 11 and 13),
- 42-year-old patients with somatoform disorders, $N = 80$ (sample 03),
- 49-year-old patients with rheumatic diseases, $N = 89$ (sample 04),
- 55-year-old patients with cardiac diseases, $N = 223$ (sample 02).

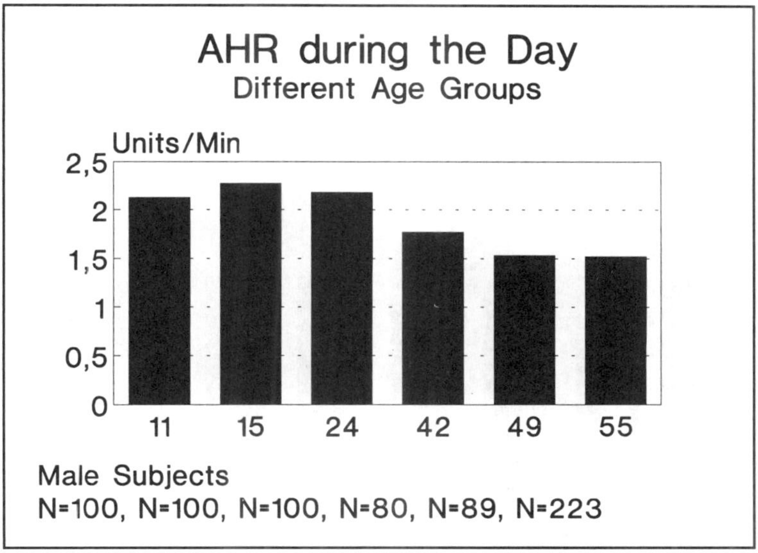

Figure 10. Additional heart rate during the day for different age groups.

As shown in Figure 10, AHR is higher during the day in the younger groups and gradually declines with increasing age. Because emotional situations might be different in students as compared with the patient samples, the course of AHR might be more valid at night (see Figure 11).

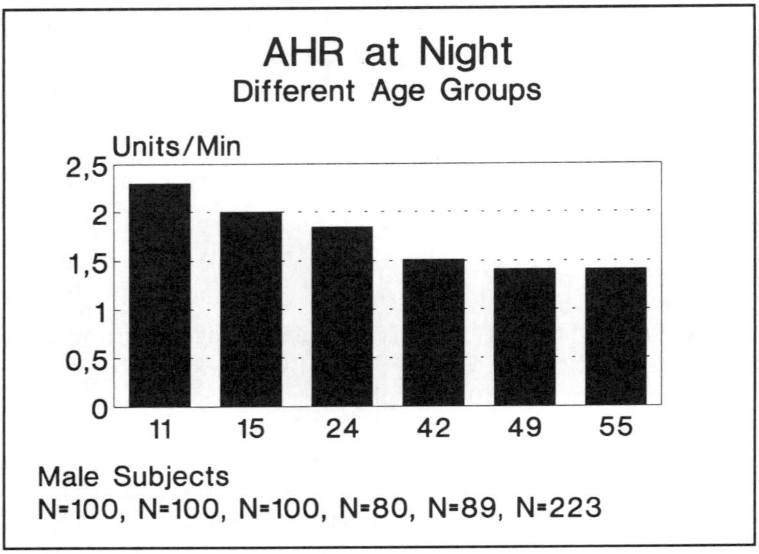

Figure 11. Additional heart rate at night for different age groups.

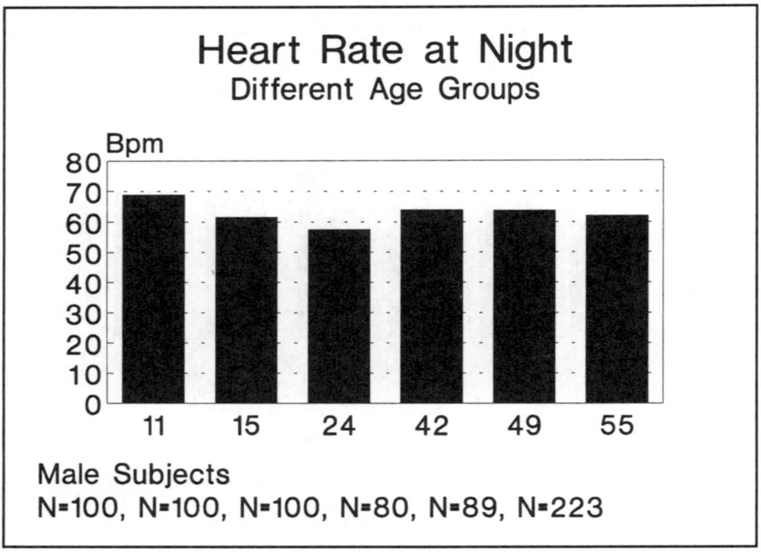

Figure 12. Heart rate at night for different age groups.

Indeed, the attenuation of AHR is more prominent during night. We can assume that AHR during the night is caused by the phases of rapid eye movements (REM) during which heart rate increases without an increase in physical activity. This attenuation, however, is not a function of heart rate itself. Figure 12 shows that heart rate at night is lowest in the 15-year-old and 24-year-old samples, whereas the patient samples show no clear cut differences. The lower heart rate in the younger samples is presumably caused by physical training effects. As we might expect, the highest heart rate at night is seen in the 11-year-old boys. This result mirrors the well-known fact that heart rate decreases from birth to at least young adulthood.

3.5.3 AHR: Emotional or mental work load?

3.5.3.1 Reaction time paradigm

Presumably, AHR is also influenced by mental work load. In a study with N = 60 male students (mean age 24.1 years), experimental load was varied with a special reaction time paradigm (Myrtek, Dieterle, & Brügner, 1990). Each item of the task consisted of 36 two-digit numbers presented in a matrix of six rows and six columns with a personal computer. Subjects had to detect the combination in which the numbers 43 and 63 occurred in the matrix and then press one of four buttons. Four combinations of equal probability could occur: 43 only, 63 only, 43 and 63, and neither 43 nor 63 (Kuhmann, Lachnit, & Vaitl, 1985). Subjects were instructed to react as quickly and correctly as possible. For individual standardization, the presentation time of the matrices was controlled by the performance of the subjects using an algorithm which adapted the presentation times according to a preset success criterion.

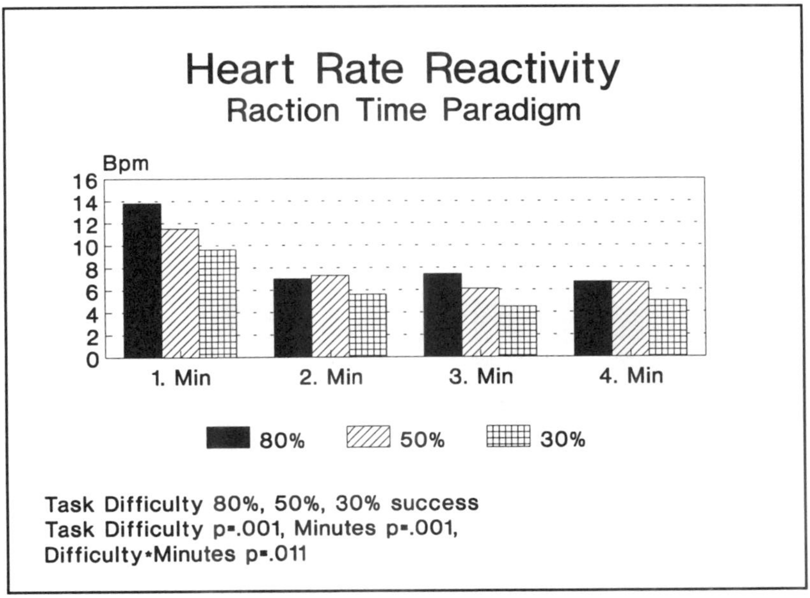

Figure 13. Heart rate reactivity during a reaction time paradigm with different task difficulties. From Myrtek et al., 1990; modified. Reproduced with permission. Copyright 1990 by the Federation of European Psychophysiology Societies.

Task difficulty was monitored by the computer with predefined levels of 80%, 50%, and 30% success or correct reactions. Each correct reaction increased a monetary bonus and each wrong or late reaction decreased this bonus. As shown in Figure 13, a progressive decrease in heart rate reactivity (differences to the preceding rest level) during continued performance at each task difficulty level could be observed.

We can assume that the reactivity in the first minute would have caused an AHR but not in the following minutes. The task was a mixture of mental work load and emotional work load because subjects won or lost money. It is obvious, however, that at the beginning of a mental task heart rate increases and may produce an AHR.

3.5.3.2 Reciting a neutral text or discussing an emotional theme

In a study with $N = 120$ male students (mean age 23.5 years; sample 10) monitoring was conducted in the laboratory during the discussion of relevant themes such as unemployment, abortion, etc. in triplets consisting of two subjects and the student experimenter (Lacher, 1994). Subjects in this experiment were paired in such a way that they would have highly different viewpoints of the discussion theme. This pairing was done by a self-rating of the opinions subjects held in a session preceding the experiment. The experiment consisted of a 30 minute discussion of the theme, reading a neutral text aloud for two minutes, viewing a section of the movie "Some like it hot" for 30 minutes, and a resting phase of four minutes. Time base of monitoring was set to four seconds with a minimal heart rate increase of six bpm to produce an AHR. Therefore, AHR values are not comparable to other AHR values of our studies which used a one minute time base. In the same way another experiment was conducted with 30 couples (mean age 40.0; sample 15; Lacher, 1997).

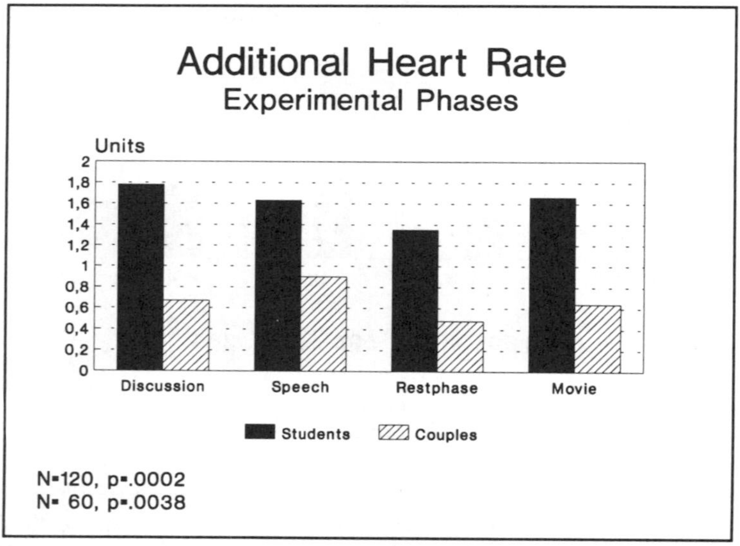

Figure 14. Additional heart rate during different experimental phases.

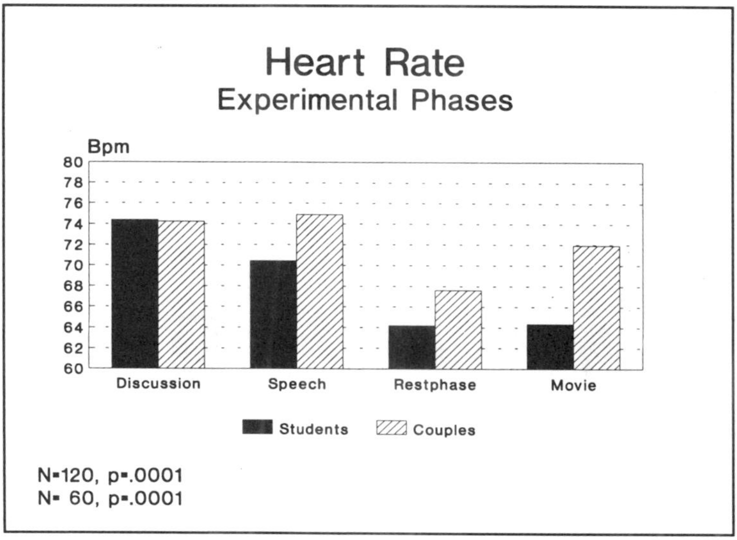

Figure 15. Heart rate during different experimental phases.

Due to the age difference of the samples, the older couples generally show lower values for AHR. During the discussion (see Figure 14), AHR was in the same range than during the recital of a neutral text or during the movie in both samples. Compared to the restphase, AHR during the discussion, the recital, and the movie was higher (*t* test for dependent samples: students $p < .001$, $p = .005$, $p < .001$; couples $p = .014$, $p < .001$, $p = .050$). In couples AHR during the recital was higher than during the movie ($p = .044$) but not in students.

In students, heart rate (see Figure 15) during the discussion was significantly different from the heart rates during the recital, the restphase, and the movie (all *p* values < .001); in couples, only the differences between discussion and restphase as well as discussion and movie are significant (all *p* values < .001). This is due to the difference in physical activity during the recital (see Figure 16). Heart rate during the recital was significantly different from heart rate during the restphase or during the movie in both samples (all *p* values < .001). In students, restphase and movie did not differ but heart rate during the movie was higher than during rest in couples ($p < .001$). The higher heart rate of the couples during the movie obviously was caused by the content of the movies. Students saw a funny movie whereas the couples were confronted with a movie about mariage problems which may well have been more relevant for them. The difference between the movies is also mirrored by physical activity because students were laughing during the funny movie. Therefore, activity was higher during the movie as compared to recital or restphase in students (both *p* values < .001).

In couples, physical activity during the recital was higher than during the movie ($p = .049$) or the restphase ($p < .001$). Finally, physical activity was highest during the discussion compared to the other phases in both samples (all *p* values < .001).

Speech activity (see Figure 17) was significantly different between all experimental phases and for both samples (all p values < .001).

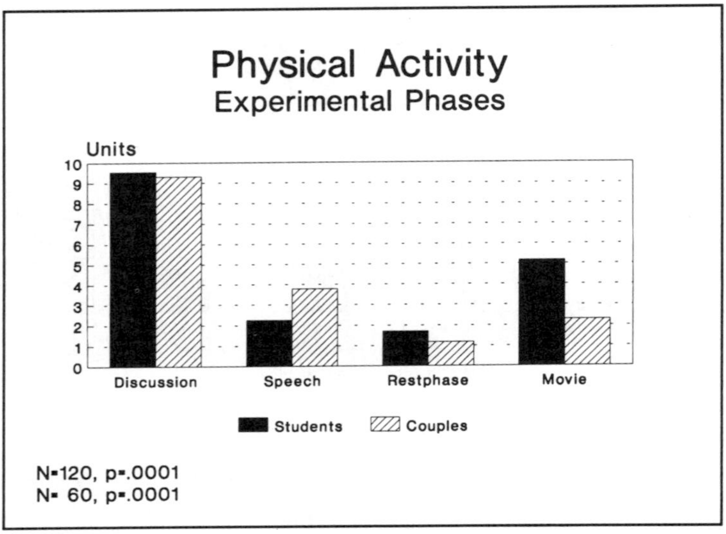

Figure 16. Physical activity during different experimental phases.

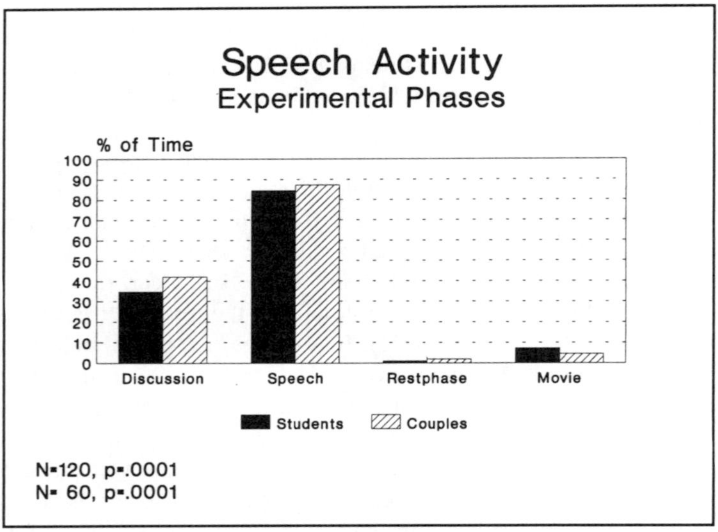

Figure 17. Speech activity during different experimental phases.

We can assume that both situations, discussion and recital, comprise a mixture of emotional and mental work load. The cognitive processing of the written words of the spoken text is primarily a mental work load. On the other hand, reading the text in the presence of other persons also has an emotional component. Discussion of a relevant theme has a mental and emotional component, too. Processing the right arguments is a mental task; but at the same time, the subject is emotionally aroused by the arguments of his counterpart.

3.6 Discussion

The main advantage of the FMS is the rather simple recording technique because only heart rate and physical activity have to be recorded. Compared to other biosignals, both parameters can be measured nearly without any artifact. Moreover, the subjects are not hampered by the equipment and not aware of the measurement itself. Both parameters, heart rate and physical activity, are able to differentiate over a wide range of physiological activation.

It could be demonstrated that the short-term reliability of the parameters heart rate, ST segment, and P-wave amplitude are high. As expected, physical activity shows only a low reliability. Medium reliabilities are observed for MSSD which may be caused by the specific sample of the reliability study. Long-term reliabilities or stability coefficients were in the same range as the short-term coefficients. The stabilities of heart rate were even higher than those derived from laboratory studies. For the longer segments such as 23h, day, and night, long-term stabilities were also computed for AHR (see Table. 3). These stabilities are fairly high, indicating that emotional reactivity seems to be a characteristic feature for the single subjects.

Most important is the validity of our emotional, mental, and physical work load components. The within-subject correlations have shown that physical activity and heart rate are actually correlated to a high degree. This is a relevant prerequisite for the decomposition of heart rate in a physical and emotional component. AHR is not correlated with physical activity and MSSD; only a small correlation exists with heart rate. According to the within-subject correlations we can conclude that physical activity is a valid indicator of the physical work load component. The correlations of AHR with the other parameters show that AHR is not a redundant parameter.

The induction of emotional arousal in laboratory experiments with different movies shows that AHR captures emotional work load. During the erotic movie as compared to the funny movie, AHR is significantly higher in both experimental conditions (sitting in a chair or working on a bicycle ergometer). Monitoring of AHR during the movie "The silence of the lambs" also points in the expected direction. AHR is higher in those passages of the film which are especially suspenseful. The correlation of AHR with some subjective ratings made for the emotional impact of the film reveals that AHR is higher in those subjects who rate the film as frightening and suspenseful.

Further validating results for the FMS come from the testing of hypotheses of expected differences between certain segments monitored under everyday life conditions. Daytime versus nighttime segments showed the expected differences for heart rate, physical activity, MSSD, and P-wave amplitude. The same was true for the comparison sitting versus standing versus walking. Heart rate, physical activity, and P-wave amplitude showed a gradually and highly significant increase from sitting to standing and to walking. The hypotheses for working time as compared to leisure time were substantiated for heart rate, physical activity, and P-wave amplitude but not for MSSD. It was hypothesized that staying at school or staying at the university as compared to staying at home will show lower MSSD and higher P-wave amplitude at the former. Both hypothesis were confirmed.

AHR was tested using social contacts with differing degree of familiarity. It was postulated that AHR and heart rate would be higher in social contacts with strangers as compared to contacts with peers and MSSD would be lower. All hypotheses were confirmed. Finally, it was postulated that the amount of TV consumption will have an effect on AHR and heart rate whereby higher consumption will show lower AHR and lower heart rate due to habituation. Meta-analyses revealed that both hypotheses are significantly confirmed.

We have considered some other aspects of AHR which might be helpful to elucidate this new parameter. AHR is normally distributed, a prerequisite for parametric statistics. Interestingly, AHR shows an age dependency which is most pronounced during the night. This dependency is not caused by heart rate itself. The result implies that the emotional reactivity is attenuated with increasing age.

A relevant question pertains to the meaning of AHR. Is AHR only an indicator of emotional work load or does AHR also mirror mental work load? We have tried to answer the question with two laboratory experiments. From the first experiment with the reaction time paradigm it is obvious that the first minute of the task would have produced an AHR. However, the reaction time paradigm comprised both mental and emotional work load. In the second experiment with discussions of emotional relevant themes, AHR was slightly higher during the discussion than during the recital of a neutral text. Here too, both situations are a mixture of emotional and mental work load. Therefore, it seems not to be possible to disentangle emotional and mental work load entirely.

MSSD offer to a certain degree the possibility to measure mental work load. This parameter is practically uncorrelated with AHR and has demonstrated some validation in our hypotheses testing. However, there is a substantial correlation with heart rate, with higher heart rate resulting in diminished MSSD. Given this fact, a firm conclusion that a decrease of the MSSD indicates mental work load can only be drawn when heart rate shows the same level in the situations compared. If heart rate is different in the situations compared, it is necessary to introduce heart rate as a covariate in the statistical tests. Mostly, a significant difference for MSSD vanishes, as observed in our studies.

P-wave amplitude is an indicator of sympathetic activation, as proven by the present results. Therefore, this parameter might be valuable for field studies. For stress-strain research, however, no new information is given by this parameter and, therefore, it can be omitted in studies of this kind.

Taken all together, we might conclude that AHR is a valid indicator of emotional and mental work load. We have also demonstrated that physical activity assessed by the device is an indicator of the physical work load component. Finally, it was demonstrated that heart rate variability, at least to a certain degree, is an indicator of mental work load.

However, minor disadvantages in the assessment of the emotional work load component should be mentioned. Increases in heart rate due to emotional factors accompanied by increasing physical activity cannot be assessed with this method. Moreover, different emotions are accompanied by various heart rate increases, resulting in the fact that emotions with stronger increases of heart rate are assessed more easily (Caprara et al., 1987; Eisenberg et al., 1988).

3.7 Summary

Heart rate is both an indicator of emotional arousal and an indicator of physical activity. As shown by several studies dealing with the issue of multiple stressors, heart rate reactivity elicited by a stressor combination is nearly an additive combination of the respective reactivity elicited by the single stressors. Therefore, it is possible to separate the emotional and physical component if physical activity reflecting the energetic demand can be measured accurately. With a special ambulatory monitoring device consisting of a small computer, this problem was solved. Heart rate and physical activity, recorded with motion detectors, are compared on-line with the device. If heart rate of a specific minute exceeds the rate of the previous minutes without an accompanying increase of physical activity, an emotional event (additional heart rate, AHR) may be assumed. In such a case, the subject is requested by a beep signal to answer relevant questions given on the display of the device of how he or she feels, about what he or she is doing, etc.

In order to assess the validity of the new method, several samples comprising about 500 subjects were used: White and blue collar workers, train and bus drivers, railway dispatchers, schoolboys as well as female and male students. Furthermore, laboratory experiments in which emotional arousal was induced by movies served to validate the AHR. The results show that heart rate is an indicator of total work load, physical activity an indicator of the physical work load component, heart rate variability (MSSD) an indicator of the mental, and AHR an indicator of the emotional work load component. P-wave amplitude was identified as a general indicator of sympathetic activation.

Chapter 4

Interoception

Interoception means the perception of bodily sensations such as hunger, thirst, tiredness, chest pain, palpitations of the heart, and so on. Some of these sensations are interpreted by the individual as indicating a disease which may lead one to search for medical advice. Other terms in this context are introspection (Mechanic & Hansell, 1987) and symptom awareness. There are individual differences in introspection resulting in different awareness and reports of bodily complaints. Several studies dealt with interoception, especially with the perception of heart rate. These studies are of theoretical interest because they can answer the question to what extent internal physiological processes can be perceived.

Symptom awareness has medical consequences as shown, for example, for the results of cardiac catheterization. About one quarter of all catheterizations show negative angiographic findings. On the other hand, one quarter of catheterizations are made too late with severe positive angiographic results. According to Frasure-Smith (1987), the latter group of patients has a low level of bodily awareness or has not complained enough about symptoms which would have led to an earlier angiography. Men with negative angiographic findings had a high level of bodily awareness whereas men with increasing positive findings had decreasing awareness.

Pennebaker (1982) has shown that bodily symptoms are perceived in the same way as external events. Because information processing is limited, external and internal sensory data compete for processing. The probability of reporting symptoms is inversely related to the quantity of external information at any given time and, therefore, dependent on the actual situational circumstances. A second important fact is that symptoms are interpreted within *cognitive schemas* or hypotheses available to the individual. According to such hypotheses, attention is directed selectively to that sensory information which supports the present hypothesis. In the opinion of Pennebaker, people are not able to perceive physiological states reliably because the interindividual and intraindividual correlations between symptoms and physiological states are typically low. Moreover, persons who perceive a special physiological state rather well, are not able to perceive another physiological state with the same accuracy. Finally, only *changes* but not the level of a physiological state are perceived.

4.1 Some findings from the literature

Several experimental studies investigated the interoception of physiological functions, especially heart rate and blood pressure. The reason for these studies is the idea that interoception might be helpful to improve the therapy of physiological disorders such as hypertension, increased resistance in the respiratory tract, arrhythmias, etc. If it is basically possible to perceive physiological functions, it would offer the opportunity to increase interoception by adequate training.

In a study by Jones, Jones, Cunningham, and Caldwell (1985), the perception of heart rate in myocardial infarction patients as compared to healthy persons was investigated. No difference in interoception between the groups was found and interoception in both groups was low. A low level of interoception was also seen in students by Katkin, Morell, Goldband, Bernstein, and Wise (1982) and by Pennebaker and Hoover (1984). Schandry (1981) investigated the accuracy of heart rate perception and the degree of emotional lability in a group of healthy persons. Emotionally labile persons showed a better perception than emotionally stable persons. The author suggests that the higher anxiety level in emotionally labile persons might be a result of their better perception of physiological functions. On the other hand, it might be that emotionally labile persons have a higher awareness of bodily functions, thus being better trained in discriminative tasks assessing the accuracy of perception. Actually, it has been shown that heart rate perception can be trained to a certain degree (Katkin et al., 1982; Weitkunat, Schandry, Sparrer, & Beck, 1987).

According to Schandry, Bestler, and Montoya (1993), interoception of heart rate is mediated by cardiodynamic parameters. The authors varied the cardiac performance of their students systematically by changing bicycle ergometric exercise on a tilt table with changing tilt angles. Stroke volume, heart rate and other parameters were assessed by impedance cardiography. Heart beat perception was dependent on body position with better perception during lying than during standing. With increasing ergometric exercise, heart beat perception was better, too. The quotient of stroke volume and left ventricular ejection time revealed the highest correlation with the accuracy of heart beat perception. It was concluded from this study that mechanoreceptors and pressoreceptors in the close vicinity of the heart are the source for cardiac perception. However, a more recent study by Ring, Liu, and Brener (1994) failed to replicate these results.

In studies of this kind the question is relevant whether the correlation between a measured physiological parameter and the same parameter estimated by the subject actually reflects an interoception or symptom awareness. It also can be that the correlation is only a conclusion of the subject, based on the present situational circumstances. Subjects will rightly suppose an increase of heart rate with increasing exercise which might falsely be interpreted as an increase in the accuracy of interoception. Ring and Brener (1996) investigated the knowledge of their subjects concerning heart rate during different body positions and during physical activity with questionnaires. In subsequent laboratory experiments, heart rate was manipulated by tilting and ergometric exercise and subjects rated their heart rates in the different settings. All heart rates (knowledge based, rated, and actual) were correlated. Rated heart rates were on average closer to the knowledge based heart rates than to the actually measured heart rates. Regression analyses revealed that the rated heart rates ("interoception") were significantly predicted both by the actually measured heart rates and by the knowledge based heart rates.

Windmann, Schonecke, Fröhlig, and Maldenar (1999) conducted an especially relevant experiment in 50 patients with cardiac pacemakers. Heart rates were set to a low (60 bpm), medium (75 bpm), and high (110 bpm) pacing rate unknown to the patients while they performed a heart beat tracking task according to the method proposed by Schandry (1981). Counting of heart rate did not follow the shifts in their actual heart rates adequately, whereby actual heart rates were systematically underestimated: 52 bpm in the low, 54 bpm in the medium, and 59 bpm in the high pacing rate. With increasing actual heart rate, differences between the actual and the estimated heart rates became higher. Only 26% of the patients perceived the heart rate manipulation and only 6% perceived that their heart rate was higher than 100 bpm during the high pacing rate. The authors conclude that tracking scores reflect beliefs about heart rates rather than cardiac sensitivity.

Similar findings were observed for the perception of blood pressure. Fahrenberg, Franck, Baas, and Jost (1995) investigated the correlations between estimated and actually measured blood pressure in patients with hypertension and normotensive controls using ambulatory blood pressure monitoring. Both groups did not show significant correlations between estimated and measured blood pressure values. However, estimated blood pressure values were significantly correlated with actual heart rate and physical activity measured with motion detectors. Even higher correlations were observed between estimated blood pressure on the one hand and physical tension and subjective physical activity on the other. It was concluded that blood pressure awareness is not a matter of perception but influenced by situational circumstances.

4.2 Cardiac perception in healthy subjects

According to the literature we can expect the following results:

- Interoception of bodily functions is low or non existent.
- Perceived symptoms are influenced by cognitive schemas.
- There are no observed differences in interoception between healthy persons and patients.

4.2.1 Perception of AHR in healthy subjects

As described in Chapter 3, feedbacks are given to the subjects as true feedbacks (AHR, heart rate increase due to emotional/mental factors) and random feedbacks (no heart rate increase due to emotional/mental factors) in order to prompt the subjects to reveal their subjective state. If subjects are able to discern these feedbacks (interoception) we would expect differences in their subjective state. With each feedback, subjects are asked to disclose their subjective state. Our expectation is that subjects are more aroused during true feedback as compared to random feedback. The second rating "enjoyment of the present situation" is not as clear. AHR should be observed during pleasant as well as during unpleasant situations. However, AHR is more pronounced for emotionally negative situations such as anger or anxiety. Therefore, the probability for a higher unpleasantness rating might be greater during true feedback with AHR.

Table 18. Mean comparisons between true and random feedback for healthy samples. Partly from Myrtek, 1998a and Myrtek & Brügner, 1996, modified. Reproduced with permission. Copyright 1998 by Huber, Bern and 1996 by Elsevier, Oxford.

Sample	Variables	True	Random	*p*
Schoolboys, 11 years	Heart rate (bpm)	96.85	91.69	**.000**
N = 100, sample 06	Physical activity (units/min)	29.13	30.47	.179
	Excitement (4=excited)	1.28	1.26	.287
	Enjoyment (5=unpleasant)	2.11	2.08	.353
Schoolboys, 15 years	Heart rate (bpm)	90.31	86.41	**.000**
N = 100, sample 07	Physical activity (units/min)	24.91	28.70	**.000**
	Excitement (4=excited)	1.35	1.34	.769
	Enjoyment (5=unpleasant)	2.24	2.23	.450
Female students	Heart rate (bpm)	90.74	84.87	**.000**
N = 50, sample 08	Physical activity (units/min)	24.48	27.35	**.037**
	Excitement (4=excited)	1.23	1.20	.157
	Enjoyment (5=unpleasant)	2.31	2.29	.558
Female students	Heart rate (bpm)	91.65	86.06	**.000**
N = 50, sample 12	Physical activity (units/min)	22.40	22.19	.841
	Excitement (4=excited)	1.31	1.28	.136
	Enjoyment (5=unpleasant)	2.43	2.35	**.009**
Male students	Heart rate (bpm)	83.32	78.33	**.001**
N = 96, sample 09	Physical activity (units/min)	23.31	25.76	**.004**
	Excitement (4=excited)	1.38	1.37	.573
	Enjoyment (5=unpleasant)	2.35	2.32	.203
Male Students	Heart rate (bpm)	85.48	81.28	**.001**
N = 50, Sample 11	Physical activity (units/min)	21.88	25.99	**.000**
	Excitement (4=excited)	1.30	1.27	.097
	Enjoyment (5=unpleasant)	2.41	2.36	.188
Male students	Heart rate (bpm)	82.22	79.04	**.000**
N = 50, sample 13	Physical activity (units/min)	18.91	22.75	**.017**
	Excitement (4=excited)	1.38	1.36	.155
	Enjoyment (5=unpleasant)	2.40	2.37	.363
Railway employees	Heart rate (bpm)	88.81	82.92	**.001**
N = 49, sample 16	Physical activity (units/min)	23.85	24.67	.580
	Excitement (4=excited)	1.15	1.15	.912
	Enjoyment (5=unpleasant)	1.93	1.90	.465
Blue/white collar workers	Heart rate (bpm)	83.64	79.03	**.000**
N = 106, sample 17	Physical activity (units/min)	23.82	27.52	**.000**
	Excitement (4=excited)	1.21	1.20	.753
	Enjoyment (5=unpleasant)	2.07	2.05	.381

Table 18 presents the mean comparisons between true and random feedback for our healthy subjects. All minutes with AHR (true feedback) were averaged for each subject. The same was done for minutes with random feedback (no indication of AHR). Statistical analysis was applied to these means using the *t* test for dependent samples. AHR is not displayed in the table because this variable is the criterion and therefore highly significant.

Heart rate is highly significant between the conditions of true and random feedback in all samples, with true feedback showing the higher heart rate. Significant differences also emerge for physical activity in six of the nine samples but here, physical activity is lower for the true feedback condition. This means that the AHR increase is very pronounced, with higher heart rate accompanied even by lower physical activity. Numerically all ratings of excitement and enjoyment are in the expected direction, but only the enjoyment rating in one female student group (sample 12) is significant. Therefore, we can confirm the first hypothesis that the interoception of heart rate is low or non existent.

4.2.2 The influence of cognitive schemas on perception

In Chapter 3.4.2 we have already briefly described our laboratory experiment with a funny and an erotic movie. The erotic movie was edited in a way that scenes with erotic content (from late night television) alternated with unequivocally pornographic scenes (from a video-tape library). Altogether the movie showed 16 minutes of erotic and 14 minutes of pornographic content. During the experimental session, the male subjects were prompted every minute by a beeper to rate their excitement for the last minute with the help of an "emotion lever" with five steps from 1 = not excited to 5 = very excited. In Table 19 the means for the two groups (rest and ergometric exercise) are taken together ($N = 96$, sample 09).

Table 19. Mean comparisons (*t* test for dependent samples) between the erotic and the pornographic sections of the movie. From Myrtek, 1998a. Reproduced with per-mission. Copyright 1998 by Huber, Bern.

Variables	Erotic	Porno	*p*
Heart rate (bpm)	71.97	71.12	.000
Physical activity (units/min)	26.98	26.66	.044
AHR (units/min)	2.62	1.79	.002
Heart rate MSSD (8.3 ms)	6.29	6.08	.004
P–wave amplitude (microV)	128.41	123.49	.000
Excitement "emotion lever"	2.70	3.20	.000

Table 19 reveals that during the erotic part as compared to the pornographic part, subjects had a significantly higher heart rate, higher physical activity, higher AHR, and higher P-wave amplitude. This means that the emotionally induced physiological arousal was clearly higher during the erotic part of the movie than during the pornographic. Heart rate variability (MSSD) was lower in the pornographic section indicating higher mental load. The physiological arousal contrasted with the subjective excitement of the students. The pornographic part of the movie was rated more exciting than the erotic part.

This result suggests a cognitive schema held by the students. We understand the paradox when we analyze the content of both movie sections. The pornographic scenes were rather hard and played by professional actors. Compared to the pornographic part, the erotic scenes were more indirect and the actors were younger. It is obvious that the students rated their excitement according to the explosiveness of the content on the basis of a cognitive schema and not by interoception. We assume that the "social distance" between the students and the girls acting in the erotic part of the movie was smaller than in the pornographic part. It was easier to develop more sympathy for the girls in the erotic part. Therefore, the second hypothesis that the perceived excitement is influenced by cognitive schemas can be confirmed. Cognitive schemas not only weaken the correlation between physiological arousal and subjective state but even convert the correlation to the opposite as demonstrated by our results.

In this context another finding is of interest. We analyzed the possible influence of the minimal physical load induced by the ergometer on the excitement rating measured by the emotion lever. As already described in Chapter 3.4.2, half of the subjects ($N = 48$) watched the movies sitting in a chair and the other half ($N = 48$) worked on a bicycle ergometer with a minimal load. In the rest condition subjects rated the excitement induced by the funny movie with a mean of 1.95 and in the erotic movie with 2.76. The respective figures for the ergometric exercise condition are 2.08 and 3.11. We conducted a two-factorial MANOVA with the factors movie (funny vs. erotic) and conditions (rest vs. exercise). The main effect for the factor movie was $F(1, 94) = 126.3$ ($p < .0001$) and for the factor condition $F(1, 94) = 5.0$ ($p = .0285$) with no significant interaction effect $F(1, 94) = 1.9$ ($p = .1737$). When we analyze the conditions for each movie apart, the funny movie yields $F(1, 94) = 1.1$ ($p = .2898$) and the erotic movie $F(1, 94) = 5.5$ ($p = .0207$).

The result of a significant condition main effect clearly denotes a transfer of excitation. Arousal induced by ergometric exercise is misattributed to arousal induced by the erotic stimuli (Cantor, Zillmann, & Bryant, 1975). Misattribution of this kind also distorts the relation between physiological symptoms and subjective state.

4.3 Cardiac perception in patients

4.3.1 Perception of AHR in patients

The third hypothesis deals with a possible difference in interoception between healthy persons and patients. According to the literature cited, one would not expect a substantial difference. Table 20 presents the mean comparisons between true and random feedback. The results are very similar to those seen in healthy subjects. Because the sample with cardiac diseases is large the small differences in the means for excitement and enjoyment become significant. Compared to the patients with somatoform disorders and patients with rheumatic diseases, heart rate in patients with cardiac diseases is low. This is due to the medication with beta-blockers in the cardiac patients. We may conclude that the perception of AHR in patients is not different from the perception in healthy subjects.

Table 20. Mean comparisons between true and random feedback for patient samples. Partly from Myrtek, 1998a and Myrtek & Brügner, 1996, modified. Reproduced with permission. Copyright 1998 by Huber, Bern and 1996 by Elsevier, Oxford.

Sample	Variables	True	Random	*p*
Cardiac diseases	Heart rate (bpm)	79.34	72.99	**.001**
N = 223, sample 02	Physical activity (units/min)	25.12	23.37	**.018**
	Excitement (4=excited)	1.19	1.16	**.020**
	Enjoyment (5=unpleasant)	2.01	1.98	**.024**
Somatoform disorders	Heart rate (bpm)	89.78	82.83	**.000**
N = 80, sample 03	Physical activity (units/min)	29.32	29.62	.786
	Excitement (4=excited)	1.37	1.34	.069
	Enjoyment (5=unpleasant)	1.97	1.97	.939
Rheumatic diseases	Heart rate (bpm)	86.83	81.83	**.000**
N = 89, sample 04	Physical activity (units/min)	24.6	30.23	**.000**
	Excitement (4=excited)	1.20	1.18	.081
	Enjoyment (5=unpleasant)	1.80	1.78	.204

4.3.2 Asymptomatic and symptomatic myocardial infarction

Myocardial infarction patients with no pain during infarction and thereafter ("silent" myocardial infarction) are an interesting group, relevant for the issue of interoception. It is known that only one third of clinically substantial ST-segment depression is accompanied by anginal pain (Freeman & Nixon, 1987; Stern et al., 1988). For the explanation of the phenomenon of asymptomatic myocardial infarction, several medical hypotheses have been suggested. First, it has been argued that a blockade of afferent cardiac nerves (e.g., by peripheral neuropathies such as diabetes mellitus) or a destruction of these nerves by the infarction might by the reason (Ambepityia et al., 1990; Cohn, 1989). Second, it was suggested that these patients exhibit a better pain inhibition by endogenous opioids than symptomatic patients (Falcone et al., 1988). Third, there might be differences in the severity of the myocardial infarction whereby the severity is greater for the symptomatic patients. Our own hypothesis is that there might be differences in the psychological status and in cognitive schemas between both groups (Myrtek, Fichtler, König, Brügner, & Müller, 1994).

From the sample with cardiac diseases (sample 02), 35 patients with no cardiac pain at the time of infarction and during the last two weeks before admission to the study were identified by questionnaire (asymptomatic myocardial infarction patients, AMI). The infarction of these patients had to be not more than three months prior to the study. Out of the remaining group, 35 MI patients who complained of pain during infarction and during the last two weeks were matched according to age and time of infarction (symptomatic myocardial infarction patients, SMI).

Clinical characteristics were assessed at the beginning of the patients'stay in the rehabilitation clinic such as site of infarct, biochemical, and hematological variables. ECG was monitored at rest, during ergometric exercise, and during Holter monitoring to assess arrhythmias. A few days after these measurements, patients were asked to fill out questionnaires to assess socioeconomic variables (housing conditions, education level, number of children, etc.), life habits (sports, consumption of cigarettes, alcohol, and tablets such as sleeping tablets, analgesics, and tranquilizers) anamnestic data (former hospital stays, premonitory symptoms, etc.), and personality traits. For the assessment of personality traits the following inventories were used: Freiburg Personality Inventory (FPI) with the scales Achievement motivation, Health concern, Extraversion, and Neuroticism (Fahrenberg, Hampel, & Selg, 1984); Life Satisfaction Questionnaire (FLZ) with the scales Health satisfaction and Work satisfaction (Fahrenberg, Myrtek, Schumacher, & Brähler, 2000); and Freiburg Complaint List (FBL) with the scale General state of health (Fahrenberg, 1994). Frequency of heart pain and sleep disturbances were rated on 5step scales. In addition, patients were monitored with the Freiburg Monitoring System (FMS) for 23 hours. At the end of the rehabilitation stay patients underwent an ergometric exercise test.

There were no significant differences between the groups in age (AMI = 54.8, SMI = 55.3 years), body weight, and height. Results of coronary angiography performed before admission to the rehabilitation clinic were available for 12 AMI and 17 SMI patients. The number of stenosed coronary arteries > 70% and the localization of the infarction were not different. Basic biochemical data such as blood status, blood sedimentation rate, blood sugar, cholesterol, triglycerides, uric acid, creatinine, calcium, potassium, sodium, etc., also showed no differences between the groups. ECG measurements during Holter monitoring (number of ventricular premature contractions, number of ventricular beat morphologies, etc.) revealed no differences either. The socioeconomic data and life habits, too, revealed no differences.

Table 21 shows the anamnestic data. Previous nursing home or hospital admissions, for any reason, and operations for any disorder, were significantly less frequent in AMI patients. SMI patients had more frequent and longer premonitory symptoms than AMI patients.

Table 21. Mean comparisons between AMI and SMI patients for anamnestic data. From Myrtek, 1998a and Myrtek et al., 1994, modified. Reproduced with permission. Copyright 1998 by Huber, Bern and 1994 by The European Society of Cardiology.

Variables	Dimension	AMI	SMI	*p*
Former hospital stays	number	2.00	3.00	.076
Former stays at nursing homes	number	0.71	2.31	**.001**
Former operations	number	1.00	1.62	**.040**
Visits to the doctor last year	number	6.00	6.71	.684
Premonitory symptoms	% of patients	33.33	67.65	**.004**
Duration of premonitory symptoms	1–5, 5=long	2.54	3.40	**.031**

Monitoring with the FMS (see Table 22) shows that physical activity throughout the day was higher for AMI patients. Despite this finding, heart rate in patients with AMI was numerically lower. Therefore, physical fitness of the SMI patients might be somewhat lower. AMI patients showed significantly more premature contractions during monitoring. This finding is also confirmed by the ergometric exercise test at the end of the rehabilitation period (Tab. 24). Especially relevant are the number and the magnitude of ST-depression episodes. No differences between the groups emerged. Interestingly, the groups showed significant differences in their subjective state during monitoring. These ratings are means based on about 45 feedbacks throughout the day. SMI patients significantly stated that they were more aroused, enjoyed their actual situation less, and perceived more heart pain than the AMI patients.

Table 22. Mean comparisons between AMI and SMI patients for variables during monitoring with the FMS. From Myrtek, 1998a and Myrtek et al., 1994, modified. Reproduced with permission. Copyright 1998 by Huber, Bern and 1994 by The European Society of Cardiology.

Variables	Dimension	AMI	SMI	*p*
Heart rate	bpm	70.1	71.5	.461
Physical activity	units/min	16.8	13.7	**.023**
AHR	units/min	1.3	1.6	.181
Ventricular premature contractions	number/hour	8.5	2.3	**.011**
ST-depression episodes	number/hour	17.7	17.2	.920
ST depression mean duration	min	6.8	5.7	.724
ST depression mean amplitude	microV	−114.5	−123.2	.167
Excitement	1–4, 4=excited	1.13	1.25	**.017**
Enjoyment	1–5, 5=unpleasant	1.86	2.05	**.041**
Heart pain	1–3, 3=strong	1.02	1.12	**.001**

Table 23. Mean comparisons between AMI and SMI patients for personality traits and physical complaints. From Myrtek, 1998a and Myrtek et al., 1994, modified. Reproduced with permission. Copyright 1998 by Huber, Bern and 1994 by The European Society of Cardiology.

Variables	Dimension	AMI	SMI	*p*
FPI Achievement motivation	0–12, 12=motivated	7.34	7.82	.488
FPI Health concern	0–12, 12=concerned	6.25	5.67	.356
FPI Extraversion	0–14, 14=extraverted	7.08	5.73	.077
FPI Neuroticism	0–14, 14=neurotic	4.94	6.70	**.029**
FLZ Health satisfaction	5–25, 25=dissatisfied	11.82	14.17	**.003**
FLZ Work satisfaction	5–25, 25=dissatisfied	9.74	10.45	.288
FBL General state of health	8–40, 40=bad	16.85	22.17	**.001**
Frequency of heart pain	1–5, 5=often	1.00	3.40	**.000**
Sleep disturbances	1–5, 5=no	3.80	3.08	**.046**

The results for personality traits and physical complaints assessed by questionnaire also point in the same direction (see Table 23). SMI patients show significantly more neuroticism and more dissatisfaction with their health. They also reveal a tendency for more introversion than the AMI patients. General complaints such as loss of appetite, dizziness, being sensitive to changings in the weather, etc., are more frequent in SMI than AMI patients. The same is true for heart pain and sleep disturbances.

At the end of the rehabilitation treatment, patients underwent an ergometric exercise test (see Table 24). No differences were observed for submaximal and maximal blood pressure and heart rate. Maximal performance was better for the AMI than for the SMI patients. However, we have to take into account that the SMI patients did not reach their maximal performance due to complaints of angina pectoris. Moreover, we have already stated that physical fitness might be better for the AMI patients.

Table 24. Mean comparisons between AMI and SMI patients for ergometric exercise variables at the end of the rehabilitation period. From Myrtek, 1998a, modified. Reproduced with permission. Copyright 1998 by Huber, Bern.

Variables	Dimension	AMI	SMI	*p*
Systolic blood pressure 50 watt	mmHg	138.3	144.6	.141
Diastolic blood pressure 50 watt	mmHg	83.2	83.4	.916
Heart rate 50 watt	bpm	87.2	91.4	.144
Systolic blood pressure max watt	mmHg	172.1	171.8	.950
Diastolic blood pressure max watt	mmHg	94.7	91.3	.183
Heart rate max watt	bpm	114.5	110.6	.302
Maximal performance	watt	111.4	94.1	**.020**
Max performance reached	1=yes, 2=no	1.18	1.38	.070
Arrhythmias during exercise	1=yes, 2=no	1.79	1.94	.067
Angina pectoris ergom exercise	0=no, 1=yes	0.39	0.88	**.014**

4.3.3 Discussion of the AMI and SMI results

On the basis of the present findings, the hypothesis that the severity of the MI or of myocardial ischemia might explain the differences in anginal pain between AMI and SMI patients is not supported. There were no differences between the groups in the number of ischemic episodes, the duration of the episodes, the depression of the ST-segment amplitude, and the number of stenosed coronary arteries. On the other hand, AMI patients showed more ventricular premature contractions than did the SMI patients. SMI patients showed lower physical activity throughout the day during monitoring. We have already stated that SMI patients reveal lower physical fitness than AMI patients. It seems that SMI patients generally have more anxiety with regard to physical exertion.

SMI patients had more frequent premonitory symptoms and these were of longer duration at the time of infarction. It might be suggested that premonitory symptoms are related to more severe coronary artery disease. Rissanen, Romo, and Siltanen (1978), however, did not find a correlation between the occurrence of premonitory symptoms and autopsy findings of coronary arteries. Likewise, in the study by Wink, Bödicker, and Kaufmann (1983) premonitory symptoms did not correlate with prognosis in MI patients.

The most important result of this study is the striking difference between the AMI and SMI groups in the psychological factors. SMI patients complained of poor health in general, were dissatisfied with their health, revealed higher neuroticism, were more introverted, and showed more pessimism as revealed in the subjective ratings during ambulatory monitoring. It is obvious that the two groups demonstrate different illness behavior. According to Mechanic (1962), *illness behavior* denotes "the ways in which given symptoms may be differentially perceived, evaluated, and acted (or not acted) upon by different persons" (p. 189).

Although the severity of the cardiac disease is the same in both groups, SMI patients feel themselves more disabled and ill. AMI patients on the other hand underestimate the severity of their illness. These different illness behaviors also have consequences for the rehabilitation outcome. At the end of the treatment 71% of patients with AMI, but only 43% of those with SMI were judged by the physicians as fit to work ($p = .015$).

We suppose that the reasons for these inadequate illness behaviors are cognitive schemas. At the center of these schemas is the relative presence or absence of neuroticism. Neuroticism is a stable personality trait which is highly correlated with physical complaints (Costa & McCrae, 1987; Myrtek, 1984, 2000). The origin of neuroticism is not entirely clear. Education, learning processes, and perhaps genetic influences seem to be relevant. In accordance with this supposition are the significant differences between AMI and SMI patients for nursing home admissions and previous surgery. It is possible that the SMI patients due to their more frequent physical complaints utilize the health care system more often than the AMI patients. On the other hand, more frequent contacts with the health care system foster a better adoption of the sick role.

It could be argued that the psychological and behavioral differences between the AMI and SMI patients might be the result of the presence or absence of anginal pain during infarction and thereafter and not the result of cognitive schemas. There are, however, several reasons that this alternative hypothesis is unlikely. First, there are no physiological differences between the AMI and SMI patients which could explain the anginal pain. Second, we have already pointed out to the stability of personality traits such as neuroticism and physical complaints, which are unlikely to be changed in the short time which elapsed between MI and the beginning of our study (on average two months). In the Baltimore Longitudinal Study of Aging by Costa and McCrae (1985), the Cornell Medical Index, a questionnaire for physical complaints, was administered a second time to 386 men after an interval of five to eight years. The correlation between the scores for total physical complaints was $r = 0.74$ ($p < .001$). The stability of neuroticism in other longitudinal studies covering 10 and 12 years was about $r = 0.70$. Third, AMI and SMI patients already show differences in previous illnesses not related to the present disease. Fourth, there are no significant correlations between personality factors and physiological variables as shown in meta-analyses (Myrtek, 1998b). Finally, there is a known association between neuroticism and future angina pectoris (Myrtek, 2000). All arguments considered, we may conclude that the presence of certain cognitive schemas is the reason for the differences observed in AMI and SMI patients. This also means that the presence or absence of anginal pain is no secure indicator of underlying coronary heart disease.

4.3.4 Emotional arousal, ischemic episodes, and angina pectoris

Several laboratory studies with patients suffering from coronary heart disease (CHD) suggest an adverse influence of emotional or mental arousal on ECG parameters such as myocardial ischemia (Burg, Jain, Soufer, Kerns, & Zaret, 1993; Gottdiener et al., 1994; Jain, Burg, Soufer, & Zaret, 1995) or ventricular arrhythmia (Freed, Thomas, Lynch, Stein, & Friedmann, 1989; Thomas et al., 1992). However, whether laboratory studies can be generalized to everyday life is a point of controversy. In recent years, some studies used ambulatory monitoring of ECG parameters and diaries to record physiological changes and patients' ratings of subjective emotional/mental stress.

As we have stated in the foregoing sections, however, subjective reports are influenced by subjects' own hypotheses or schemas. Therefore, reports of subjective stress are often independent of the physiological status as pointed out in Chapter 4.3.2. Moreover, physical and emotional activities were mostly confounded in the studies cited above, making a clear interpretation difficult. With the FMS using AHR it is possible to disentangle the effects of the physical and emotional activity, because emotional arousal can be assessed independently of the subjective reports (Myrtek, Frölich, Fichtler, & Brügner, 2000).

Of the 223 CHD patients (sample 02), 49 patients with ischemic episodes during waking hours were identified and 115 patients had ventricular premature contractions (VPCs) during monitoring. Mean age of the first group was 54.8 and of the second group 55.9 years. There was an overlap of 27 patients between both groups that means that these patients had ischemic episodes and VPCs during the time of observation. Ischemic episodes were operationalized as described in Chapter 3.1.5.3. Analysis of VPCs was carried out visually for each 20th minute of the whole record (waking hours) plus the minutes with feedbacks. Here, only the number of VPCs is considered because most VPCs were isolated VPCs. Multivariate comparisons between ischemic episodes or VPCs and control minutes were done with the generalized T^2 statistic (Hotelling's T^2; Anderson, 1984), followed by univariate t tests for dependent samples. Wilks's Lambda was used to determine the F values.

As indicated in Table 25, AHR was significantly higher during ischemic episodes than during control periods. Physical activity and heart rate were higher during these episodes, too. This is in accordance with findings by Gullette et al. (1997) and Rehman, Zalos, Andrews, Mulcahy, and Quyyumi (1997). During ischemic minutes, VPCs were not more frequent than during control periods. Thirty patients received feedback during ischemic and control periods. There were no differences in ratings of heart pain, excitement or enjoyment of the actual situation.

Table 25. Mean comparisons between minutes with ischemic episodes versus control minutes without ischemic episodes. From Myrtek et al., 2000, modified. Reproduced with permission. Copyright 2000 by the Federation of European Psychophysiology Societies.

Variable	Dimension	N	Control	Episodes	*p*
Minutes record length	number	49	73.63	62.47	.557
Physical activity	units/min	49	22.73	41.74	**.001**
Heart rate	bpm	49	73.08	85.40	**.001**
AHR	units/min	49	1.64	3.94	**.005**
ST amplitude	microV	49	–45.03	–118.25	**.001**
VPCs	number/hour	49	0.14	0.09	.509
Excitement	1–4, 4=excited	30	1.18	1.21	.679
Enjoyment	1–5, 5=unpleasant	30	1.95	1.92	.807
Heart pain	1–3, 3=strong	30	1.15	1.18	.771

Generalized T^2 statistic for physiological parameters: $F(5, 44) = 44.72, p = .0001$.
Generalized T^2 statistic for psychological parameters: $F(3, 27) = 0.14, p = .9355$.

Of the 223 CHD patients, 115 (52%) revealed minutes with VCPs with a mean of 9.7 VPCs/h (see Table 26). There was no significant difference in AHR during minutes with VPCs as opposed to control minutes. The figures for AHR in Table 26 are higher than in Table 25 because all feedback minutes where included in the analysis of VPCs (more than half of these minutes were minutes with AHR). Heart rate was significantly higher during minutes with VPCs but physical activity showed no difference. As stated already for the ischemic episodes, there was no association between VPCs and ischemia (ST amplitude 100 ms after the R wave, ST depression > 100 microV). The psychological parameters also revealed no significant differences.

Table 26. Mean comparisons between minutes with ventricular premature contractions (VPCs) versus control minutes without VPCs. From Myrtek et al., 2000, modified. Reproduced with permission. Copyright 2000 by the Federation of European Psychophysiology Societies.

Variable	Dimension	*N*	Control	VPCs	*p*
Minutes record length	number	115	74.81	9.01	**.001**
Physical activity	units/min	115	23.50	24.45	.635
Heart rate	bpm	115	74.05	76.32	**.008**
AHR	units/min	115	4.61	4.70	.828
ST amplitude	microV	115	–3.96	–5.19	.426
VPCs	number/hour	115	0.00	9.71	**.001**
ST depr > 100 microV	number/min	115	0.02	0.02	.741
Excitement	1–4, 4=excited	97	1.14	1.15	.644
Enjoyment	1–5, 5=unpleasant	97	1.99	1.95	.418
Heart pain	1–3, 3=strong	97	1.05	1.03	.235

Generalized T^2 statistic for physiological parameters: $F(6, 109) = 49.18, p = .0001$.
Generalized T^2 statistic for psychological parameters: $F(3, 94) = 1.09, p = .3590$.

Our hypothesis that emotional or mental arousal has an adverse influence on ECG parameters is partly confirmed. Emotional/mental arousal as operationalized by AHR was associated with ischemia but not with arrhythmia. Ischemia was associated in our study with AHR and increased physical activity with concomitant heart rate increase. AHR and physical activity act independently on ischemia because physical activity and AHR are not correlated (Chapter 3.41, Table 9). In the study by Gullette et al. (1997), physical activity and emotional arousal were independent predictors of the ischemic episodes, too. These results suggest that patients with myocardial ischemia should avoid strenuous emotional or mental situations and strong physical activity to prevent silent ischemia.

The findings in the literature concerning emotional arousal and VPCs are, however, inconsistent. Shear et al. (1987) observed in a small ambulatory monitoring study an association between VPCs and panic attacks, whereas Brenner, Oberacker, Kranig, and Buchwalsky (1993) found no association between noise episodes from military flights and VPCs. The findings of the laboratory studies are also at variance with each other. Freed et al. (1989) observed in a study with 37 coronary patients in nine patients a significant increase of ventricular arrhythmias during a talking period about their daily activities as compared to a baseline. However, no differences of ventricular arrhythmias were reported by Delle Chiaie et al. (1996) between an hour of stress exposure (Raven's progressive matrix test tables) and a control hour at the same time the following day in 18 patients with mitral valve prolapse and 20 healthy controls. In a large study with 265 myocardial infarction patients with ventricular arrhythmias, no significant correlations were found between the rate of VPCs and several psychological factors (state anxiety, anger, depression) or stress reactivity to a video game (Follick et al., 1990).

In our study we found no association between ischemia and arrhythmia. This corresponds to a study by Currie and Saltissi (1993) who did not find an association between ventricular arrhythmias after myocardial infarction and transient myocardial ischemia during daily activities in 201 patients. Quyyumi et al. (1986) found in only two of 74 CHD patients an association between ST-segment change and ventricular tachycardia during ST segment monitoring.

Another result of our study is especially important for the issue of interoception. Both ischemia and arrhythmia were not associated with heart pain, rating of excitement, and rating of the pleasantness of the actual situation. Likewise, in the study conducted by Gullette et al. (1997) only 2% of the 388 ischemic episodes were associated with anginal pain. These findings are in line with our study on asymptomatic and symptomatic MI and other studies on silent ischemia (Barry et al., 1988; Cohn, 1989; Freeman, Nixon, Sallabank, & Reaveley, 1987). The absence of an association between ischemia and heart pain has serious consequences for the detection of CHD patients as well as their treatment and rehabilitation. Detection of CHD has to rely on medical examinations because anginal pain is not unequivocally related to objective cardiac events.

4.3.5 Interoception in patients with cardiac neurosis and controls

According to Schandry (1981), emotionally labile healthy persons showed a better heart rate perception than emotionally stable persons. We will test this hypothesis again with our sample of predominantly somatoform disorders (sample 03). Patients with cardiac neurosis are especially emotionally labile and should be more able to discern true from random feedbacks as compared to the other patients in this sample. It was suggested that the higher anxiety level in emotionally labile persons might be a result of their better perception of physiological functions.

Out of these patients, 38 patients were characterized by heart and thorax related symptoms without organic lesion of the heart (89% with a diagnosis of cardiac neurosis and 11% with respiratory malfunction, e.g., hyperventilation). The other 42 patients of the sample had no heart-related symptoms and served as controls. This sample comprised the following diagnoses: physiological malfunction arising from mental factors with the exclusion of the previous mentioned diagnoses (26%), depressive adjustment reaction (24%), neurotic disorders (12%), personality disorders (2%), and diverse non heart-related organic disorders (36%).

Patients were monitored with the FMS for 23 hours and filled in several psychological questionnaires: Freiburg Personality Inventory (FPI) with the scales Achievement motivation, Health concern, Extraversion, and Neuroticism, a preliminary form of the Life Satisfaction Questionnaire (FLZ) with the scales Health satisfaction and Work satisfaction, and the Freiburg Complaint List (FBL) with the scale General state of health and Cardiac complaints. In addition, socioeconomic and anamnestic data as well as living habits were recorded. Table 27 shows the characteristics of the patient samples. No significant mean differences for the socioeconomic and anamnestic data emerged.

Table 27. Mean comparisons (simple ANOVA) between patients with cardiac neurosis and control patients for socioeconomic and anamnestic data.

Variables	Dimension	*N*	Neur	N	Contr	*p*
Age	years	38	41.34	42	42.38	.618
Education level school	^=good	38	2.28	42	2.02	.179
Children	number	38	1.65	42	1.90	.384
Housing conditions	1–4, 4=good	38	3.23	42	3.09	.542
Former hospital stays	number	38	3.84	42	3.02	.217
Former stays at nursing homes	number	38	1.52	42	1.31	.485
Former operations	number	38	2.18	42	1.69	.252
Visits to the doctor last year	number	38	9.15	42	8.02	.544
Tobacco consumption	cigarettes/day	38	9.84	42	8.31	.654
Alcohol consumption	units/week	38	2.90	42	3.61	.453
Sports	units ^=active	38	25.02	42	27.14	.732

At the beginning of the rehabilitation treatment, patients underwent an ergometric exercise test (see Table 28). At the submaximal exercise level, heart rate was marginally higher for the control group and maximal performance was somewhat better for the patients with cardiac neurosis. Therefore, it can be stated that the physical fitness of the cardiac neurosis group is at least as good than the fitness of the controls.

Table 28. Mean comparisons (simple ANOVA) between patients with cardiac neurosis and control patients for ergometric exercise variables at the beginning of the rehabilitation treatment.

Variables	Dimension	*N*	Neur	*N*	Contr	*p*
Systolic blood press 100 watt	mmHg	30	173.13	20	176.00	.604
Diastolic blood press 100 watt	mmHg	30	98.83	20	96.00	.392
Heart rate 100 watt	bpm	30	115.06	20	121.50	.068
Systolic blood press max watt	mmHg	30	197.33	20	191.50	.361
Diastolic blood press max watt	mmHg	30	100.83	20	98.00	.441
Heart rate max watt	bpm	30	134.66	20	132.21	.605
Maximal performance	watt	30	146.66	20	133.75	.094
Ventricular prem contractions	0=no, 1=yes	30	0.10	20	0.15	.609
Angina pectoris	0=no, 1=yes	30	0.00	20	0.05	.222

There are striking differences evident in certain personality traits and physical complaints (seeTable 29). Patients with cardiac neurosis are indeed more emotionally labile than the other patients in this study. They are dissatisfied with their health and have more often physical complaints, especially cardiac complaints. These patients also rate their physical fitness to be lower than that of the control patients. As we have seen from Table 28, however, there is no difference in objective physical fitness between the groups. On the contrary, cardiac neurotics were physically somewhat fitter.

Table 29. Mean comparisons (simple ANOVA) between patients with cardiac neurosis and control patients for personality traits and physical complaints at the beginning of the rehabilitation treatment.

Variables	Dimension	*N*	Neur	*N*	Contr	*p*
FPI Achievement motivation	^=motivated	38	7.63	42	7.88	.702
FPI Health concern	^=concerned	38	6.10	42	7.09	.115
FPI Extraversion	^=extraverted	38	6.18	42	6.52	.679
FPI Neuroticism	^=neurotic	38	10.60	42	8.66	**.007**
FLZ Health satisfaction	^=dissatisfied	38	28.00	42	22.59	**.007**
FLZ Work satisfaction	^=dissatisfied	38	22.60	42	20.07	.174
FBL General state of health	^=dissatisfied	38	24.86	41	21.63	**.035**
FBL Cardiac complaints	^=many	37	21.16	40	15.25	**.001**
Physical fitness	^=bad	37	2.48	42	1.81	**.006**
Sleep disturbances	^=no	38	2.42	41	2.82	.193

To answer the hypothesis of a better perception of heart rate in patients with cardiac neurosis, we conducted a two-factorial MANOVA with the factor group (cardiac neurosis vs. control) and the factor condition (true feedback vs. random feedback).

As we might expect, heart rate is about seven bpm higher during true feedback as compared to random feedback with no difference for physical activity (see Table 30).

Table 30. Two-factorial MANOVA with the factors Group (*N* = 38 patients with cardiac neurosis vs. *N* = 42 control patients) and Condition (true feedback vs. random feedback).

Variable	True		Random		MANOVA		
	Neur	Control	Neur	Control	Grou	Cond	Inter
Physical activity	27.78	30.71	28.09	31.01	.145	.800	.999
Heart rate	88.05	91.35	81.45	84.08	.177	**.000**	.467
Excitement	1.45	1.29	1.42	1.26	**.009**	.075	.986
Enjoyment	2.08	1.87	2.07	1.88	**.033**	.976	.693
Heart pain	1.13	1.07	1.11	1.06	.067	.051	.660

For the dimensions of variables see Table 26.

If patients with cardiac neurosis have better interoception than controls, we would expect significant interaction effects at least for excitement and heart pain. All interaction effects are not significant. The significant group differences for excitement and enjoyment show that patients with cardiac neurosis generally rate their subjective state to be more excited and unpleasant than that of the control subjects. The nearly significant group difference for heart pain denotes that cardiac neurotics are more readily complain of angina pectoris than controls. Our hypothesis of a better perception of heart rate in patients with cardiac neurosis is thus not substantiated.

In order to study pain sensations more closely, patients were requested to activate the system by themselves if they perceived heart pain. These activations were treated like the other feedbacks from the system, i.e., the next feedback occurred between 10 and 20 minutes after the patient had initiated the system. Only eight patients, six belonging to the cardiac neurosis group and two to the control group, activated the system one or more times due to heart pain. A comparison of these pain situations with the mean of every 20th minute of the day record is made in Table 31 for the ECG and psychological variables.

Table 31. Mean comparisons (*t* test) between minutes with heart pain versus control minutes without pain for ECG parameters and subjective state.

Variable	Dimension	*N*	Pain	Control	*p*
Physical activity	units/min	8	23.74	30.02	.226
Heart rate	bpm	8	85.56	83.56	.321
ST amplitude	microV	8	–53.40	–49.05	.745
VPCs	number/hour	8	0.00	0.01	.352
Excitement	1–4, 4=excited	8	2.18	1.78	.224
Enjoyment	1–5, 5=unpleasant	8	2.84	2.35	.115
Heart pain	1–3, 3=strong	8	2.06	1.40	**.003**

Note: ST amplitude was defined in this study as a point of the ST segment lying 40% after the R wave related to the distance between R wave and T wave.

As can be seen from Table 31, all physiological variables are not significant. Of the psychological variables, heart pain rating naturally is significant and the patients rate themselves numerically to be a bit more excited whereby the actual situation is also rated as a bit more unpleasant. This finding means that patients do not perceive heart pain on the basis of physiological variables, e.g., ST-segment depression, but on the basis of situations that are more unpleasant or exciting.

4.4 Discussion

Interoception is the perception of bodily sensations. The *medical model* is at least partly based on interoception. If a person has no physical complaints this person is regarded healthy. If someone complains of angina pectoris for example, this person could have a CHD. In this case, an examination by a physician is indicated. As pointed out in the introduction of this Chapter, this perspective on things is too simple. The model does work when we have an acute impairment such as a broken bone but is insufficient when we suffer a chronic disease such as hypertension or diabetes mellitus. Evolution has created many good sensors for the perception of the relevant things in our environment. There are also a lot of sensors inside the body (e.g., mechano- and chemoreceptors) but this information is not consciously perceived. It serves for the information of the control centers in the autonomic nervous system. The information we receive from inside the body is equivocal and, therefore, open to interpretation.

We have conducted a lot of studies with healthy subjects and patients to investigate the accuracy of perception, especially the perception of heart rate. If heart rate perception were good, we might expect differences in the subjective state when comparing true feedback with random feedback. Our studies with nine different healthy samples and altogether 651 subjects showed that the ratings of excitement and enjoyment of the actual situation were numerically in the expected direction but only the enjoyment rating in one group was significant. We concluded that the interoception of heart rate was low or non existent.

As pointed out by Pennebaker (1982), bodily symptoms are interpreted within cognitive schemas or hypotheses available to the individual. This hypothesis was tested in our laboratory experiment in 96 male students with an erotic movie. Subjects rated the pornographic part of the movie to be significantly more exciting than the erotic part. However, AHR and heart rate revealed quite the opposite, whereby the erotic part was physiologically more exciting. These results are clearly indicative of the effect of a cognitive schema held by the students and of the lesser role of interoception. We also observed a transfer of excitation whereby the arousal induced by the ergometric exercise was falsely attributed to be induced by the erotic stimuli. Therefore, we may conclude that cognitive schemas can heavily distort the relation between physiological symptoms and their perception. The relevance of cognitive schemas was also shown with the comparison between asymptomatic and symptomatic myocardial infarction patients. We have already discussed these results in Chapter 4.3.3.

A third hypothesis dealt with a possible difference in interoception between healthy persons and patients. We investigated patients with cardiac diseases, with somatoform disorders, and with rheumatic diseases. No patient group was better in the perception of heart rate than the healthy groups.

Clinically relevant is the perception of heart pain. As pointed out already, the medical model is based on symptom perception. The comparison of ischemic episodes with control episodes in patients with CHD showed no difference in anginal pain. This means that the absence of angina pectoris is no indicator for a healthy heart. Therefore, medical examinations are necessary to provide information on the state of the heart.

It is also important to note that AHR is related to ST-segment depression. This is in line with studies by Barry et al. (1988), Burg et al. (1993), Gottdiener et al. (1994), Freeman et al. (1987), and Jain et al. (1995) who observed a correlation between emotional arousal and depression of the ST segment. The finding also adds to the validity of AHR as an indicator of emotional arousal.

Our last example of absent interoception pertains to patient with cardiac neurosis compared to other patients with somatoform disorders. The former group is not medically different to the latter. However, patients with cardiac neurosis are more dissatisfied with their health, emotionally more labile and have more often physical complaints. The hypothesis that these patients might have a better perception of the heart was not substantiated.

4.5 Summary

Interoception is defined as the perception of bodily sensations such as palpitations of the heart, chest pain, and so on. A proper interoception would be crucial for the *medical model.* This model suggests that a person will be regarded as healthy when physical complaints are absent. The model only works, however, during acute impairment but not in chronic diseases. Inside the body we have a lot of sensors for autonomic control but no sensors which properly inform of the state of the body. Therefore, the information from inside the body is equivocal and open to interpretation. The interpretation is dependant on situational factors, *cognitive schemas*, personality traits, and so on.

The comparison of true feedback with random feedback in several studies with healthy persons and patients has shown that all of these were not able to discern these different situations. This means that heart rate cannot be well perceived. We also observed that patients with coronary heart disease (CHD) or patients with somatoform disorders were not superior in the perception of heart rate to the healthy groups. The same was observed when we compared patients with cardiac neurosis with other patients with somatoform disorders not related to the heart. The hypothesis that the former patients might have a better perception was not substantiated. In our laboratory study with students, it was also shown that interoception is dependent on cognitive schemas. Subjects rated the pornographic part of a movie to be more exciting than the erotic part, although AHR and heart rate were significantly higher during the erotic part.

In comparing patients with an asymptomatic MI and symptomatic MI patients revealed no medical differences between both groups. However, striking differences between AMI and SMI patients were observed for psychological factors. SMI patients were emotionally more labile and showed more pessimism as revealed in the subjective ratings during ambulatory monitoring. These findings were interpreted within the context of the *inadequate illness behavior model* which is based on cognitive schemas.

We also found that the perception of heart pain is independent of the physiological state of the heart. The comparison of ischemic episodes with control episodes in patients with CHD showed no difference in anginal pain. It was concluded that the absence of angina pectoris is not an indicator for the absence of a CHD. Therefore, medical examinations are necessary to exclude a CHD. Finally, it was shown that AHR is associated with ST-segment depression. This means that emotional arousal might have adverse effects on the heart.

Chapter 5

Perception of emotions

This Chapter is based on three studies with university students (samples 12, 13, and 14). The first sample comprised 50 female students, the second 50 male students, and the last sample 40 male students. Subjects were monitored for 23 hours and asked about their emotional state directly during true and random feedbacks. In these studies, subjects did not know the nature of the feedbacks. They were only told that the feedbacks served to monitor their daily activities. In case of a perceived emotion, subjects were asked to disclose the nature of the emotion. The following emotions were listed on the display of the device: happiness, anger, anxiety/fear, sadness, surprise, and disgust. Moreover, subjects were encouraged to activate the system by themselves in order to record their psychological state when they perceived an emotion.

In the first study, a mean of 34.9 true feedbacks and of 18.6 random feedbacks was observed. The system was activated by 39 women with a mean of 2.6 activations. The second study revealed a mean of 29.8 true feedbacks and 15.8 random feedbacks. Self-activation of the system occurred in 31 students with a mean of 1.9 activations. The figures for the last study are 31.0 true feedbacks and 14.7 random feedbacks. The system was activated by 20 students with a mean of 2.3 activations.

In the studies, subjects were asked to complete the following questionnaires: German version of the State-Trait-Anger-Expression Inventory (STAXI; Schwenkmezger, Hodapp, & Spielberger, 1992), German version of the State-Trait-Anxiety Inventory (STAI; Laux, Glanzmann, Schaffner, & Spielberger, 1981), Freiburg Personality Inventory (FPI; Fahrenberg et al., 1984), and Life Satisfaction Questionnaire (FLZ; subscale "health satisfaction"; Fahrenberg et al., 2000).

Based on the findings of our studies we will answer the following questions:

- Frequency and quality of emotions;
- Possible emotional differences between true and random feedbacks;
- Physiological profiles of different emotions;
- Accuracy of the perception of emotional arousal; and
- Influence of personality dimensions on the emotions reported.

5.1 Frequency and quality of emotions

During the feedbacks, "no emotion" was reported most frequently in all samples, 58.3% in female students, 70.1% in the first male sample, and 71.6% in the second male sample. The most frequent emotion was happiness with 27.6%, 23.6%, and 19.7% followed by anger with 7.8%, 3.7%, and 4.6%, and anxiety/fear with 3.3%,

1.2%, and 1.9%, respectively. All other emotions were rare and below 2% (see Figure 18 and 19).

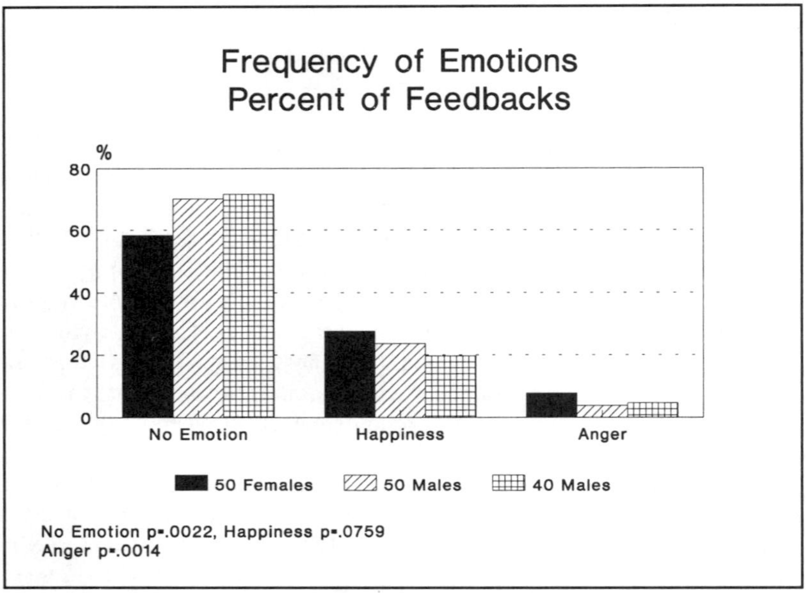

Figure 18. Frequency of "no emotion", happiness, and anger during feedbacks.

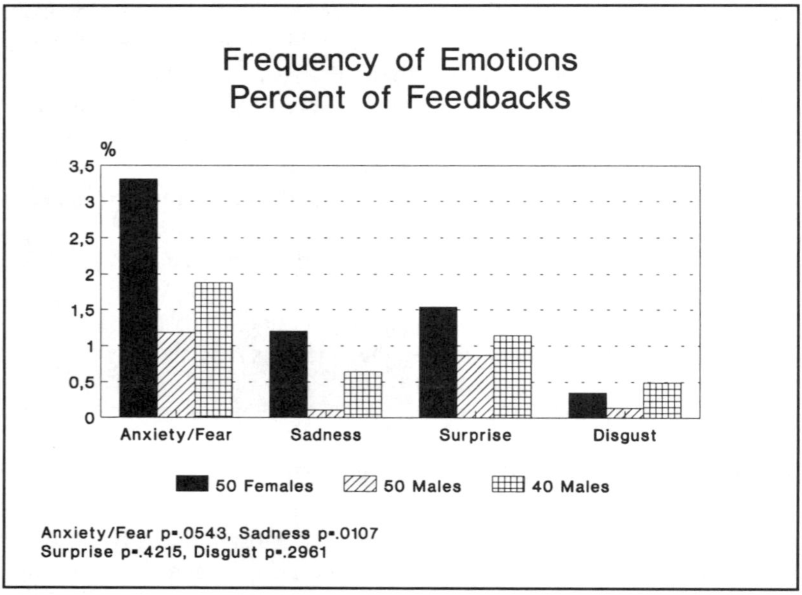

Figure 19. Frequency of anxiety/fear, sadness, surprise, and disgust during feedbacks.

Analysis of variance (ANOVA) revealed that female students reported less "no emotion" during feedbacks and, therefore, had more emotions than their male counterparts. The simple comparison between female students and male students of the first sample is significant with p = .006 and between the former and the second male sample with p = .003 with no significant difference between the male samples.

As shown in Figure 18, female students reported somewhat higher frequencies of happiness than male students, whereby the difference was significant for the second male student sample (p = .017). The difference between the male samples was not significant. The same applies for anger. Females reported anger more often than males with p = .001 and p = .017, respectively with no significant difference between the male samples. Female students also had the tendency to report anxiety/fear and sadness more often. For anxiety the difference between female students and male students of the first sample is significant (p = .011). Both male samples are not significantly different. Finally, sadness is more prominent in females with a significant difference for the first male sample (p = .003). Sadness also shows a difference between the male samples, the second sample reporting more sadness (p = .037). The other emotions, surprise and disgust reveal no sex differences.

The studies also offer the opportunity to subjectively appraise different emotions according to excitement (arousal) and affective valence, the most important emotional dimensions (Bradley, Greenwald, & Hamm, 1993; Wundt, 1905). We will confine our examination to the emotions happiness, anger, and anxiety/fear because the other emotions are too rare in occurence.

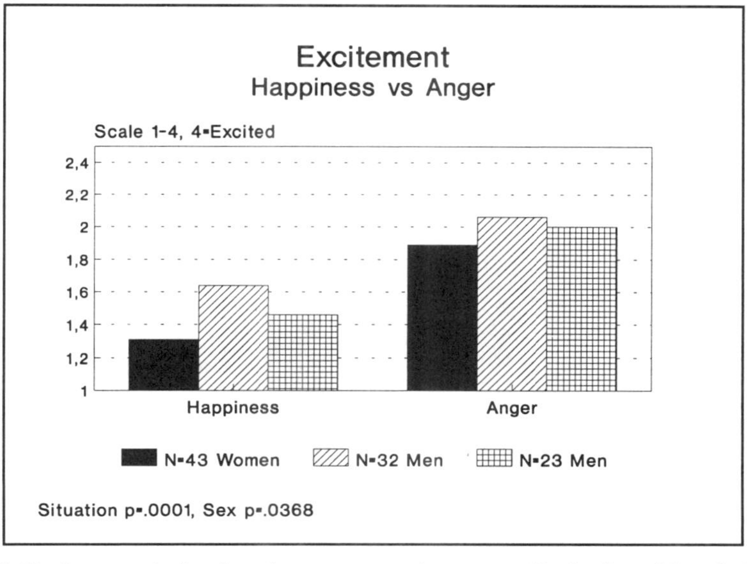

Figure 20. Excitement during happiness compared to anger. Partly from Myrtek, Zanda, & Aschenbrenner, 2001. Reproduced with permission from *Progress in Ambulatory Assessment* by Fahrenberg & Myrtek, ISBN 0-88937-225-X, p. 424. Copyright 2001 by Hogrefe & Huber Publishers, Seattle, Toronto, Göttingen, Bern.

As we can see from the Figures 20 and 21, anger is significantly more exciting and less enjoyable than happiness. The sex difference shows that males are somewhat more excited than females during both emotions.

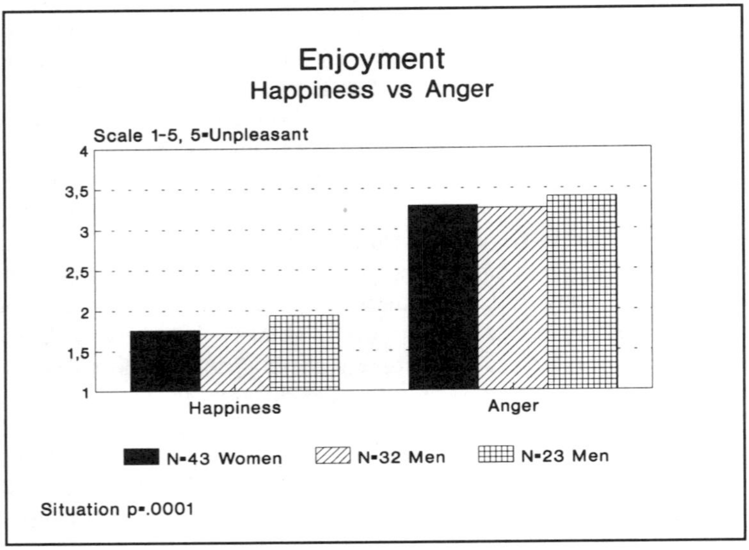

Figure 21. Enjoyment during happiness compared to anger. Partly from Myrtek et al., 2001. Reproduced with permission (see Figure 20).

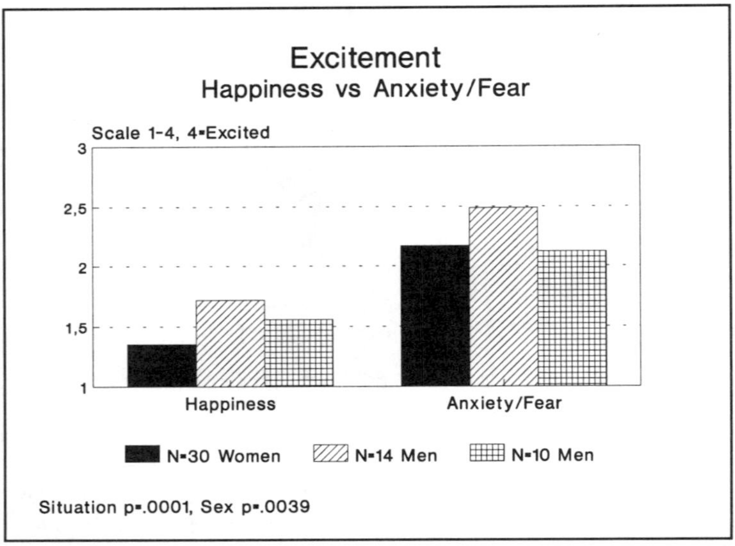

Figure 22. Excitement during happiness compared to anxiety/fear. Partly from Myrtek et al., 2001. Reproduced with permission (see Figure 20).

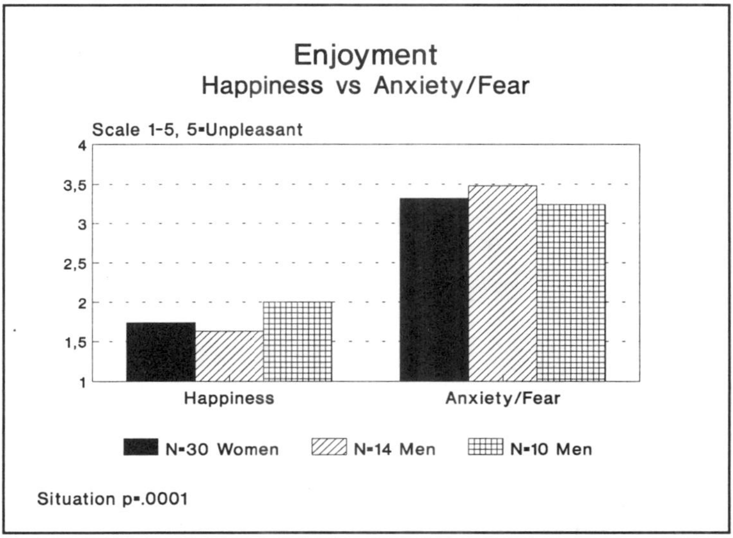

Figure 23. Enjoyment during happiness compared to anxiety/fear. Partly from Myrtek et al., 2001. Reproduced with permission (see Figure 20).

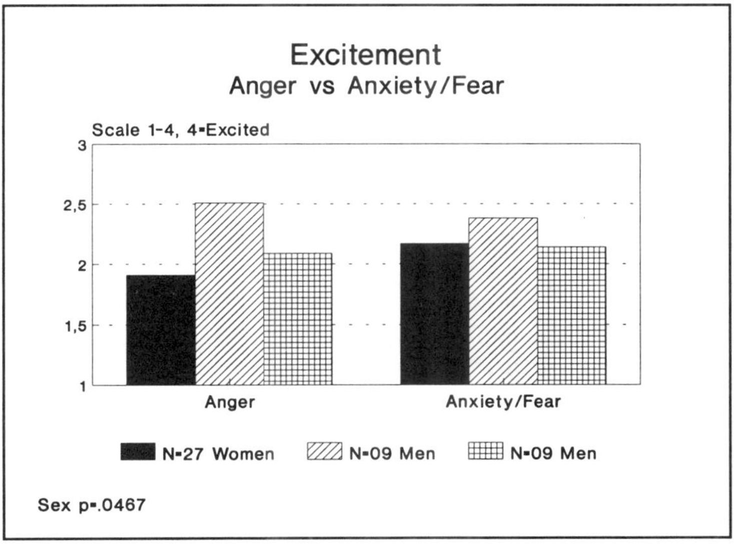

Figure 24. Excitement during anger compared to anxiety/fear. Partly from Myrtek et al., 2001. Reproduced with permission (see Figure 20).

Figures 22 and 23 show the comparison between happiness and anxiety/fear. As we might expect, anxiety/fear is more exciting and less enjoyable than happiness. Our final comparison pertains to anger and anxiety/fear (see Figures 24 and 25). There is no significant difference between the two emotions. The significant sex difference for excitement shows that male students are a little more excited than female students in both emotions. Altogether, however, we may conclude that the subjective quality of these emotions is rated as being very similar by both sexes.

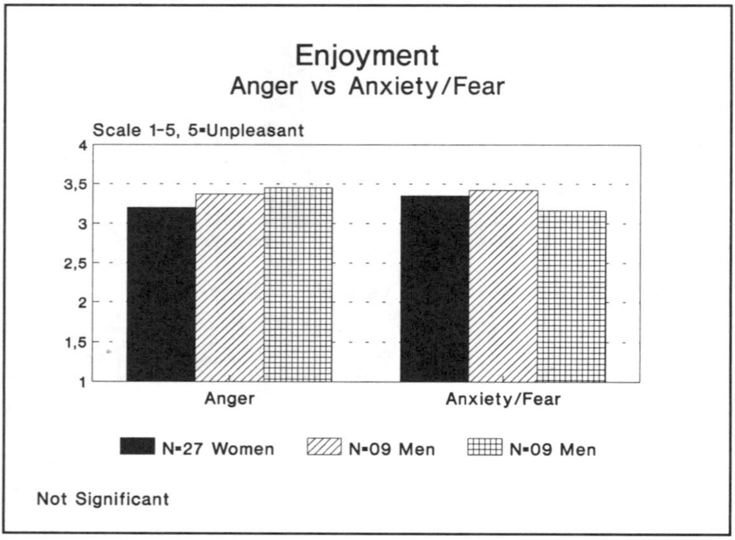

Figure 25. Enjoyment during anger compared to anxiety/fear. Partly from Myrtek et al., 2001. Reproduced with permission (see Figure 20).

5.2 Emotional differences between true and random feedbacks and for different social contacts

If emotions are based on interoception, one would expect differences between true feedback with AHR and random feedback without AHR. The frequency of emotions ought to be higher during true feedback compared to random feedback. Table 32 shows the mean values for the frequency of emotions during true and random feedback for the female and first male group. With a MANOVA the main effects "feedback" and "sex," as well as the interaction "feedback * sex" were tested.

As we can see, the main effect "feedback" is significant only for anxiety/ fear but not for the other emotions. The significant main effects for "sex" reveal the above stated fact that women report more emotions than men. All interactions "feedback * sex" are not significant. This means that women are not better than men in discerning the different physiological states associated with the presence or absence of AHR.

In these student groups we tested another hypothesis. We assumed that contacts with personal friends such as boyfriends or girlfriends are more likely to produce emotions than contacts with other students or being alone. Therefore, we analyzed these different social situations. Of the 50 female students, $N = 46$ had social contacts with personal friends and other students.

Table 32. Frequency of different emotions (% of feedbacks) during true and random feedback in 50 female and 50 male students.

Emotion	True		Random		*p*		
	Female	Male	Female	Male	Feedb	Sex	F * S
Happiness	26.4	22.0	28.2	22.9	.235	.174	.680
Anger	7.4	2.9	7.0	3.3	.992	**.000**	.515
Anxiety/Fear	3.0	1.2	2.3	0.5	**.006**	**.012**	.935
Sadness	0.8	0.1	1.7	0.1	.105	**.005**	.093
Surprise	1.3	0.8	1.5	0.5	.834	.176	.486
Disgust	0.2	0.0	0.3	0.0	.724	.212	.724

According to our expectation, perceived emotions were more frequent in the interaction with personal friends (63.7% of all feedback minutes plus the minutes with self activation) than in the interaction with other students (30.8%) or being alone (31.5%). MANOVA for social contacts (personal friends, other students, being alone) was significant with $F(2, 44) = 34.81$, $p = .0001$.

Of the 50 male students, $N = 43$ had social contacts both with personal friends and other students. Perceived emotions occurred with a frequency of 58.2% in the interaction with friends. During interactions with other students emotions were reported with a frequency of 29.7%, and being alone showed a frequency of 22.7%. MANOVA was significant with $F(2, 41) = 30.45$, $p = .0001$. We may conclude that our hypothesis is verified.

5.3 Physiological profiles of different emotions

The fact that emotions were not more frequent during true feedback compared to random feedback would suggest that reproducible physiological differences between the different emotions may not exist. We will not reprint the extensive Tables from Myrtek and coworkers (2001) but only mention the most important results.

In the studies with female students and the first male student sample, we recorded several physiological parameters: physical activity, heart rate, AHR, heart rate variability (MSSD), P-wave amplitude, ST-segment amplitude, and speech activity. Speech activity was recorded continuously with a sampling rate of 256 Hz using a small microphone attached on the larynx (% activity/ min). Multivariate comparisons between the different emotion categories were done with the generalized T^2 statistic, followed by univariate t tests for dependent samples.

Between feedback minutes without emotions and feedback minutes with emotions (including minutes with self-activation of the system) mean comparisons were drawn for the physiological parameters. Of the 50 female students, 49 reported at least a total of one minute of happiness, 43 anger, 30 anxiety/fear, 14 sadness, 17 surprise, and

6 disgust. Although the generalized T^2 statistic between minutes with and without emotions was significant for happiness and sadness, the results in the univariate analyses were disappointing. Physical activity, MSSD, and P-wave amplitude were not different between minutes with and without emotions for all of the six emotions in the univariate analyses. During surprise, heart rate was lower. AHR was even lower during happiness and sadness. Anger revealed a lower ST-segment amplitude as compared to "no emotion." Happiness was accompanied by higher speech activity. Therefore, only ST-segment amplitude and speech activity were in the expected direction.

We tried to replicate these findings in the first male student group. Of the 50 male students, 45 reported happiness, 31 anger, 12 anxiety/fear, 3 sadness, 14 surprise, and 6 disgust. The T^2 statistic was significant for happiness. In the univariate analyses speech activity only could be replicated. Here, too, speech activity was higher during happiness compared to "no emotion."

Happiness, anger, and anxiety/fear were the most frequent emotions. Therefore, we carried out mean comparisons between these three emotions, respectively. In the female sample, T^2 statistic was significant for happiness compared to anger. Minutes with anger revealed greater physical activity, higher heart rate, greater P-wave amplitude, lower ST-segment amplitude, and less speech activity than minutes with happiness. All these differences are in the expected direction. In the male students, T^2 statistic was marginally significant ($p = .098$) for happiness compared to anger, too. The univariate analyses, however, showed that only speech activity was significant, with higher speech activity during happiness. We must state that the physiological profiles for the different emotions are rather uncharacteristic and could not be replicated.

5.4 Accuracy of the perception of emotional arousal

As we have seen in Chapter 5.2, only the frequency of anxiety/fear showed a significant difference between true and random feedback. The frequency of all other emotions was not different for the feedbacks. It is possible that differences might exist between subjects' accuracy of the emotional perception, thus obscuring differences between true and random feedback. We defined accuracy as either the percentage of correctly classified true feedbacks (identification of an emotion) or random feedbacks (reporting that no emotion was present). Our hypothesis was that subjects with good emotional perception would have a high percentage of correct classifications for both true *and* random feedbacks. In this case we might expect a *positive* correlation between correctly classified true feedbacks and correctly classified random feedbacks.

Contrary to our expectations, we observed high *negative* correlations. For the female students the correlation was $r = -0.89$, for the first male group $r = -0.82$, and for the second male group $r = -0.65$. Indeed, there were high positive correlations, too, between the perception of "no emotion" during true feedback and "no emotion" during random feedback and the perception of an emotion during true and an emotion during random feedback. This finding was unexpected. We therefore, searched for other explanations. We examined the statistical distribution of both accuracy parameters, the possible statistical dependency of both parameters due to the limited number of feedbacks, and the possibility that subjects refused to answer the questions that were posed on the display correctly. All alternative explications could be ruled out.

We must conclude that two types of emotional perception exist. Obviously, there are "emotional subjects" who often perceive emotions regardless of the physiological arousal and "cool subjects" who seldom perceive emotions. Therefore, "emotional subjects" spuriously identify true feedbacks correctly but random feedbacks incorrectly, whereas "cool subjects" have a high "accuracy" rate for random feedbacks but not for true feedbacks. It is quite clear that the perception of an emotion is most likely not an interoception at all but a matter of subjects' cognitive schemas.

5.5 Influence of personality dimensions on emotions reported

Interestingly, only anxiety/fear showed consistent correlations with three personality dimensions for all samples but not happiness or anger (see Table 33). As stated in Chapter 5.2, only anxiety/fear showed a difference between true feedback compared to random feedback. The frequency of anxiety/fear was higher during true feedback. Therefore, it might be that this emotion has the greatest chance of being perceived by interoception and not only by cognitive schemas. According to Table 33, subjects who describe themselves as more anxious, more emotionally labile, and more dissatisfied with their health are more likely to perceive anxiety/fear during everyday life.

Table 33. Correlations between anxiety/fear (percent of all feedbacks) and personality dimensions in three different samples.

	Anxiety/Fear
STAI anxiety, high = anxious	**0.24**
	0.31
	0.32
FPI emotional lability, high = labile	**0.30**
	0.15
	0.30
FLZ health satisfaction, high = dissatisfied	**0.25**
	0.15
	0.36

Note: First line $N = 50$ women, second line $N = 50$ men (0.24 $p = .100$, 0.28 $p = .050$, 0.36 $p = .010$, 0.45 $p = .001$), third line $N = 40$ men (0.26 $p = .100$, 0.31 $p = .050$, 0.40 $p = .010$, 0.50 $p = .001$).

5.6 Discussion

Most of the feedbacks were not accompanied by an emotion. The most frequent emotion was happiness followed by anger and anxiety/fear. All other emotions were very rare. This is in accordance with the study by Schwartz, Warren, and Pickering (1994). These authors observed in their 24 hour blood pressure monitoring study that 65% of all blood pressure readings were neutral. Happiness was the most frequent emotion (12%), followed by anxiety (7%) and anger (1%). In a similar study by Shapiro, Jamner, and Goldstein (1997) it was observed that a happy mood was the most frequent mood in subjects' reports. Female students reported significantly more emotions than male students. This was observed especially for anger, happiness, anxiety/fear, and sadness. Between the both male samples, no systematic differences in the report of a special emotion was observed.

The most prominent qualities of an emotion are excitement and enjoyment or affective valence. In an experiment by Johnsen et al. (1995) with 96 female students using the Ekman faces, the authors reported the following equation for excitement: fear = angry > surprise > disgust = sad = happy > neutral. For pleasantness the following equation was reported: happiness > neutral > surprise > sad = fear = angry = disgust.

Because only happiness, anger, and anxiety/fear were perceived frequently in our studies, we can compare only these emotions with one another. Anger and anxiety/fear were significantly more exciting and less enjoyable than happiness but no differences between anger and anxiety/fear were observed. This is in line with the results by Johnsen et al. (1995). Males were somewhat more excited than females during both anger and anxiety/fear. It must be concluded that the subjective quality of an emotion is rated very similar by both sexes.

If we assume that emotions are based on interoception, one would expect differences in the frequency of emotions reported during true and random feedback. This hypothesis was tested in the female and first male sample. A significant difference was observed only for anxiety/fear. Obviously, in everyday life most of the emotions reported seem not to be based on interoception. We also found that perceived emotions are dependent on the situational circumstances. In both sexes, emotions were significantly more frequent during the interaction with personal friends as compared to the interaction with other students or being alone.

Our endeavour to find reproducible physiological differences between the different emotions was not successful. The physiological profiles for the emotions were uncharacteristic and could not be replicated. This finding is in accordance with other ambulatory monitoring studies. Johnston and Anastasiades (1990) conducted a study with 31 students who underwent 24 hour ECG and EMG monitoring and completed a brief mood questionnaire every 30 minutes. Time-series analysis showed that heart rate correlated with the emotional state only in very few subjects. In the study by Schwartz et al. (1994), 246 subjects were investigated with 24 hour ambulatory blood pressure monitoring. Subjects were asked to rate several moods (e.g., angry, sad, anxious, happy) in a diary each time the recorder operated. Significant increases of blood pressure were observed for angry and happy mood only after controlling for body position and location. The heart rate changes were inconsistent. The same technique was applied to 197 students in the study by Shapiro et al. (1997). Subjects who frequently reported feeling angry during the day had higher blood pressure. All other moods did not correlate with blood pressure. Heart rate showed no significant correlation at all.

According to Gray (1994), fight, active avoidance, and behavioral inhibition are mediated by three different brain systems, each of which appears to be related to a different emotional state. All these behaviors, however, require the mobilization of energy whereby the autonomic nervous system for such mobilization is triggered in much the same way in every behavior. If this statement is valid, one would not expect characteristic physiological profiles for the different emotions. The results for the physiological parameters sharply contrasted with the psychological parameters in our studies. The latter being in accordance with the perceived emotions.

The twofold replicated results on the accuracy of emotion perception deserves attention. The correlation between the percentage of correctly classified true feedbacks and the percentage of correctly classified random feedbacks was highly negative. We concluded that there are two types of emotion perception: "emotional subjects" and "cool subjects". This means that emotions reported during everyday life are often not interoceptions but based on cognitive schemas.

Several personality dispositions are related to emotions. There might be, for example, a propensity for high trait anxious persons to view uncertain events as possible threats (Frijda, 1994). Of the different emotions, only anxiety/fear showed reproducible correlations with personality dimensions. This emotion was, moreover, the only one to reveal a higher frequency during true compared to random feedback. As in the present study, Shapiro et al. (1997) reported a positive correlation between the percentage of anxious mood and trait anxiety. These authors also observed a negative correlation between happy mood and anxiety whereas anger and sadness were positively correlated with hostility.

As stated in Chapter 1, studies on emotions in everyday life have to rely as yet on self-reported emotional events assessed by diaries. Of course, subjects can report only those emotions they are aware of, leading to the question as to what extent physiological activation of emotional origin is actually perceived. As shown by Pennebaker (1982), emotion perception is not necessarily linked to physiological changes but seems essentially to be a function of cognitive schemas. With our new method we have avoided this difficulty in perception. We have detected those events with emotionally-induced physiological activation and acquired time-locked information of the subjective feeling of the individual during such events.

Indeed, emotion perception in daily life is to a great extent a function of cognitive schemas. Our results are in line with the statements made by Pennebaker (1982). They are in accordance with a review on emotion research done by Reisenzein (1983). The author concluded that peripheral arousal is no necessary condition for an emotional state as claimed by the perception model. Rimé et al. (1990) have shown that people have social schemas about peripheral changes in emotion, and that these schemata are similar across cultures. It might well be "that distinctive patterns of actual peripheral changes occur only during especially intense emotions. These extreme states could constitute exemplars or generate prototypes that would be generalized to less intense states" (p. 46). Obviously, this assumption is correct. Female and male students hold the same view regarding excitement and enjoyment during emotions such as happiness, anger, and anxiety because everybody has perceived such states in his life. However, such strong affective states are rare events and not common in everyday life. It is likely that during monitoring only a few subjects, if any, have experienced such strong affective states. Subjects infer their emotional state by external or internal cues. This assumption would explain both the missing physiological differentiation between the different emotions on the one hand and the reproducible subjective appraisal of the emotions on the other.

5.7 Summary

Three studies with university students were conducted, one with 50 female, the other with 50 male and a third sample with 40 male students. Subjects were monitored for 23 hours and asked about their emotional state directly during true and random feedbacks. When an emotion was perceived, subjects were asked to disclose what kind of emotion it was. The following emotions were listed on the display of the device: happiness, anger, anxiety/fear, sadness, surprise, and disgust.

Most of the feedbacks were not accompanied by an emotion. The most frequent emotion was happiness followed by anger and anxiety/fear. All other emotions were very rare. Female students reported significantly more emotions than male students. Between the both male samples, no systematic difference in the report of a special emotion was observed. Anger and anxiety/fear were significantly more exciting and less enjoyable than happiness but no differences between anger and anxiety/fear were observed. Both sexes rated the subjective quality of the emotions very similarly.

If emotions are based on interoception, one would expect differences in the frequency of emotions reported during true and random feedback. A significant difference was observed only for anxiety/fear. Therefore, in everyday life most of the emotions reported are not based on interoception. No reproducible physiological differences between the different emotions were found. This finding for the physiological parameters sharply contrasted with the psychological parameters in our studies which were in accordance with the perceived emotions.

It is possible that differences might exist between subjects' accuracy of emotional perception, thus obscuring differences between true and random feedback. We defined accuracy as either the percentage of correctly classified true feedbacks (identification of an emotion) or random feedbacks (reporting that no emotion was present). Therefore, subjects with good emotional perception must have a high percentage of correct classifications for both true *and* random feedbacks. In this case we might expect a *positive* correlation between correctly classified true feedbacks and correctly classified random feedbacks. However, the correlation between the percentage of correctly classified true feedbacks and the percentage of correctly classified random feedbacks was highly negative. This result was replicated twice. We concluded that there are two types of emotion perception: "emotional subjects" and "cool subjects". This means that emotions reported during everyday life are often not based on interoceptions but on cognitive schemas. Of the different emotions, only anxiety/fear showed reproducible correlations with personality dimensions. Subjects who described themselves as more anxious, more emotionally labile, and more dissatisfied with their health were more likely to perceive anxiety/fear during monitoring.

Emotion perception in daily life is to a great extent a function of cognitive schemas. Female and male students hold the same view regarding excitement and enjoyment during emotions such as happiness, anger, and anxiety because everybody has perceived such states in his life. However, such strong affective states are rare events and not common in everyday life. It is likely that during monitoring only a few subjects, if any, have experienced such strong affective states. Subjects infer their emotional state by external or internal cues. This assumption would explain both the missing physiological differentiation between the different emotions on the one hand and the reproducible subjective appraisal of the emotions on the other.

Chapter 6

Stress and strain at the workplace

6.1 Work load in train drivers, bus drivers, and dispatchers

In the following we report on studies conducted with 23 train drivers, 13 bus drivers, and 13 dispatchers with the FMS. Because it was not possible to have subjects rate their activities during work, two observers rated, in each study, subjects' special work tasks. A categorical system was developed, with each category rated every minute for approximately two working hours by two experienced observers who accompanied the subjects during work (subjects were drawn from sample 16).

6.1.1 Work load in train drivers

Twenty-three male train drivers, 12 driving a high speed train (intercity or eurocity trains between Basel/Switzerland and Frankfurt/Germany) and 11 driving a normal train on a mountain track (between Freiburg/Germany and Neustadt/Black forest; altitude difference about 700 m) with an average age of 47.0 years were studied on a normal working day (Myrtek et al., 1994). Two observers accompanied the drivers in the cabin. The following categories were used to characterize the actual work:

- Mode of driving for every minute: start, moving, change of speed, coming to a halt, standstill.
- Speed of the train for every minute: average speed during the respective minute in steps of 10 km/h.
- Stress of the situation rated for every minute by the observers: 3-step rating scale (no stress, moderate stress, high stress).
- Stress of the situation rated for every five minutes by the drivers themselves.

Compared to "moving" (see Figure 26), "start," "braking to halt," and "standstill" all showed an increase in heart rate (*t* test for dependent samples: $p < .001$, $p = .003$, $p < .001$, respectively). This cannot be explained by physical activity (see Figure 27). Physical activity was not different during "moving" and "change of speed" but both modes showed higher activity as compared to the other modes (all *p* values $< .001$). The differences in physical activity were caused by the vibration of the train and not by the physical activity of the train drivers. Figure 28 shows that AHR as compared to "moving" was higher during "braking to halt" ($p = .012$), "standstill" ($p = .002$), and "starting" ($p = .057$). No significant differences were observed for heart rate variability (see Figure 29). The stress ratings made by the observers (see Figure 30), however, were only higher for "braking to halt" as compared to "starting" ($p = .001$), "moving" ($p < .001$), "change of speed" ($p = .013$), and "standstill" ($p = .015$). Therefore, these ratings are not in line with the physiological work load indicators.

The ratings made by the drivers themselves (see Figure 31) were not significantly different for the modes of driving.

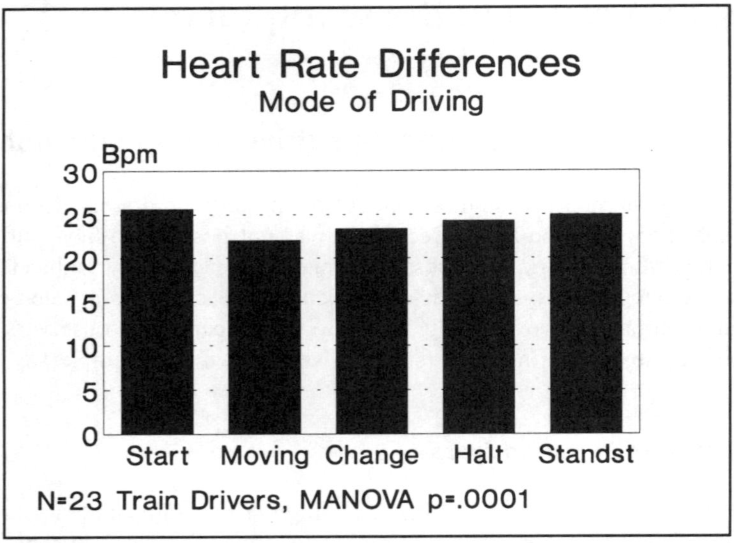

Figure 26. Heart rate (differences to baseline) in train drivers during different modes of driving. From Myrtek et al., 1994. Reproduced with permission. Copyright 1994 by Taylor & Francis, London (http://www.tandf.co.uk/).

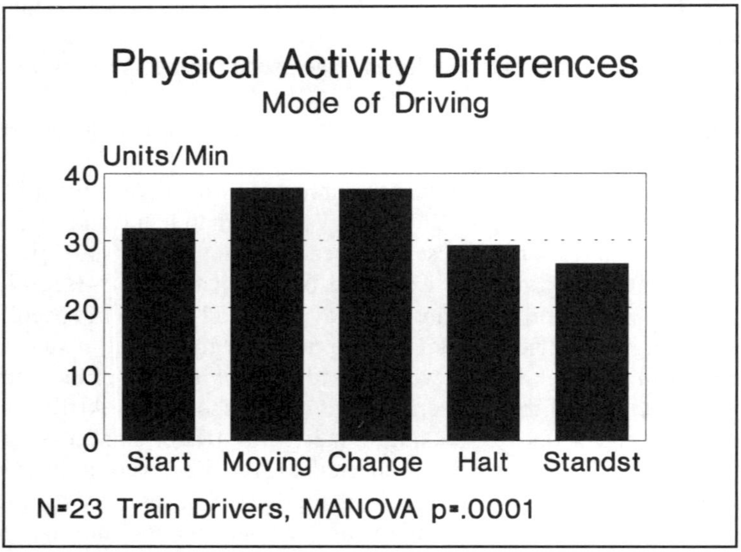

Figure 27. Physical activity (differences to baseline) in train drivers during different modes of driving. From Myrtek et al., 1994. Reproduced with permission (see Figure 26).

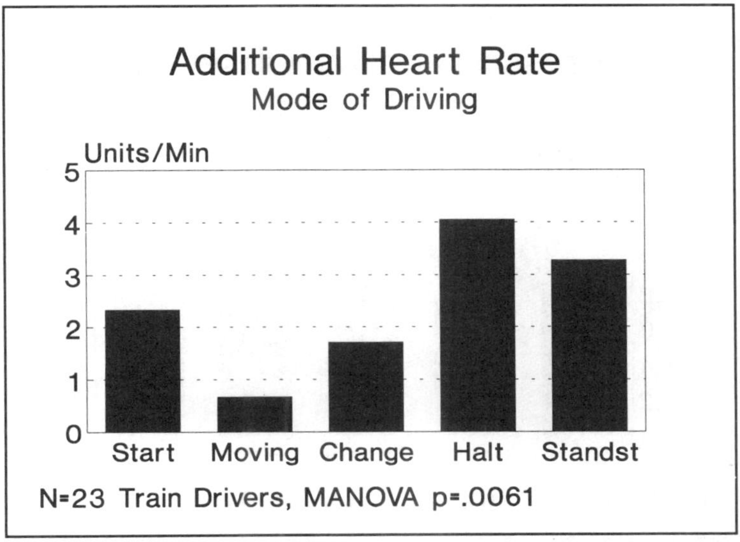

Figure 28. Additional heart rate in train drivers during different modes of driving. From Myrtek et al., 1994, modified. Reproduced with permission (see Figure 26).

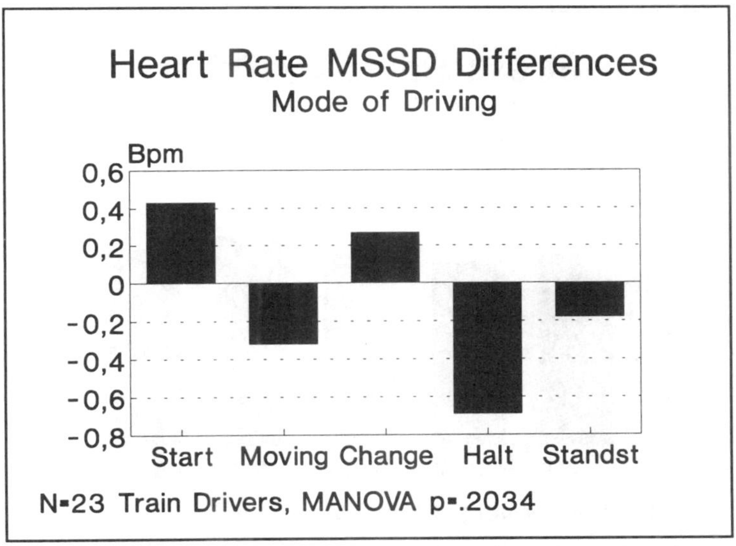

Figure 29. Heart rate variability MSSD (differences to baseline) in train drivers during different modes of driving. From Myrtek et al., 1994, modified. Reproduced with permission (see Figure 26).

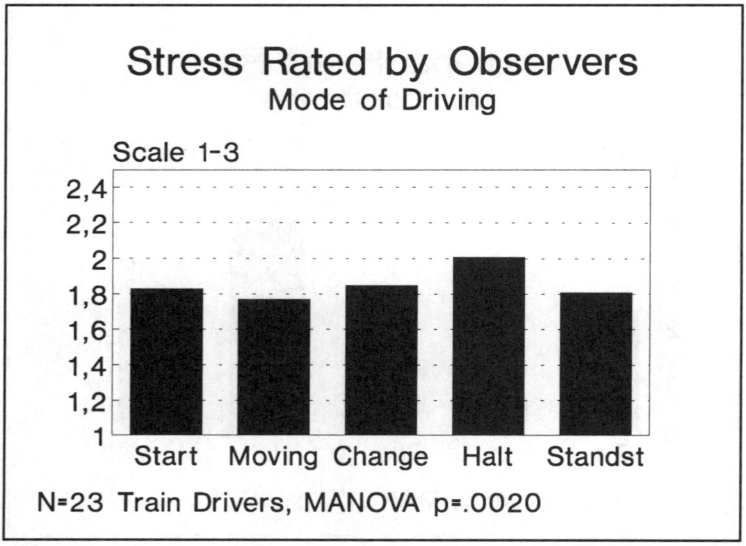

Figure 30. Stress ratings by the observers during different modes of driving. From Myrtek et al., 1994. Reproduced with permission (see Figure 26).

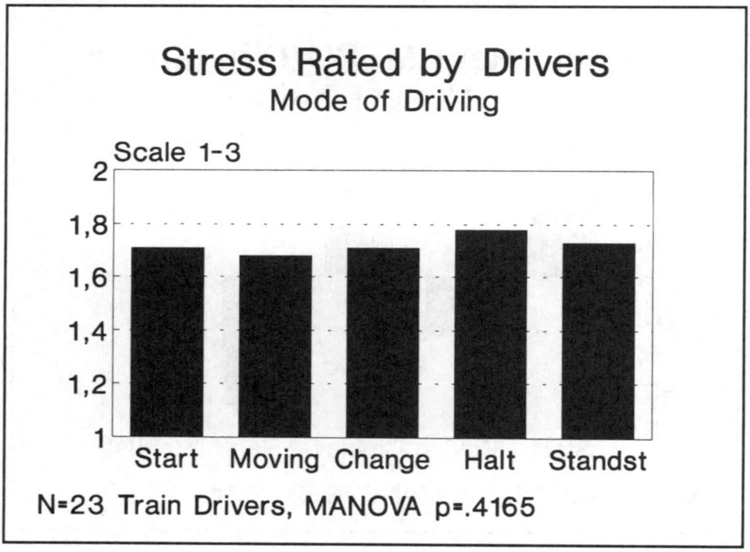

Figure 31. Stress ratings by the train drivers during different modes of driving. From Myrtek et al., 1994. Reproduced with permission (see Figure 26).

In the following, different speeds of the train are analyzed. The speed categories comprise "standstill," "speeds up to 40 km/h," "speed 40 to 60 km/h," "60 to 80 km/h," and "80 to 100 km/h." Figure 32 depicts the result for heart rate.

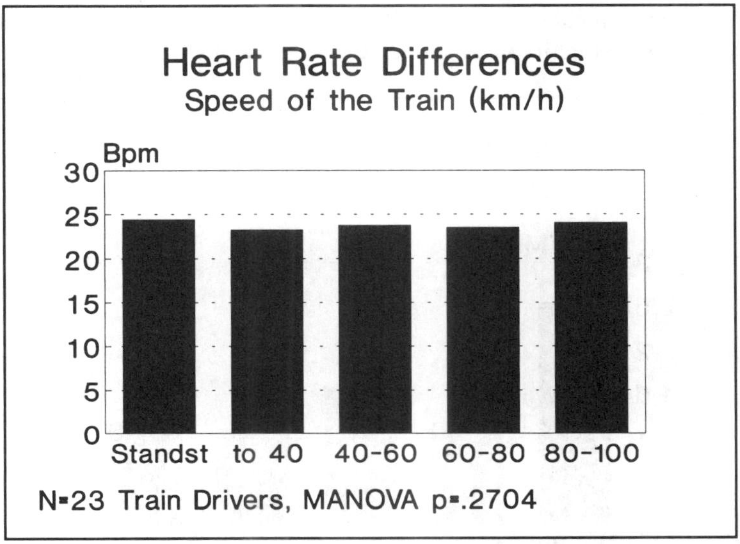

Figure 32. Heart rate (differences to baseline) in train drivers during different speeds of the train. From Myrtek et al., 1994. Reproduced with permission (see Figure 26).

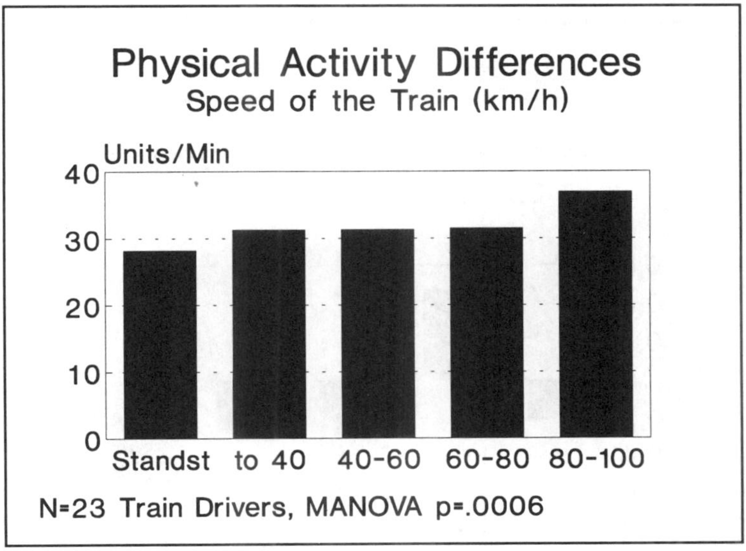

Figure 33. Physical activity (differences to baseline) in train drivers during different speeds of the train. From Myrtek et al., 1994. Reproduced with permission (see Figure 26).

No significant changes of heart rate were observed for all categories. Physical activity increased with the speed categories (see Figure 33). Compared to all other categories, activity in category "80 to 100 km/h" was highest (all p values < .001). This means that the vibrations of the engine increased with augmenting speeds.

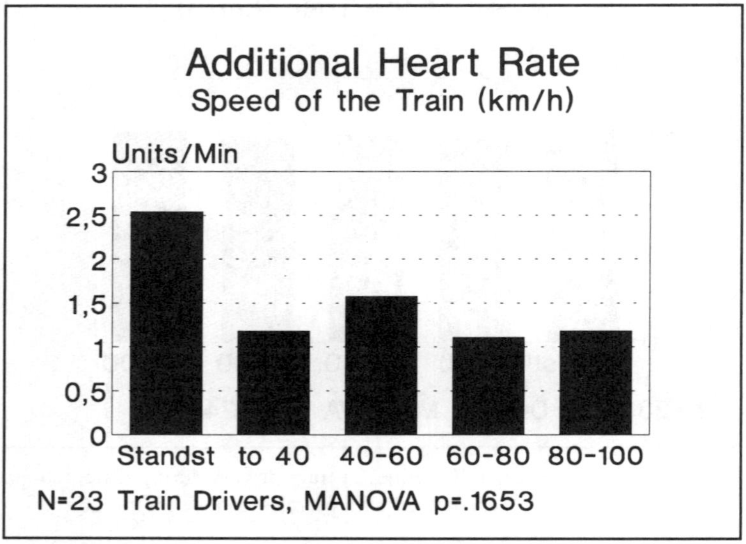

Figure 34. Additional heart rate in train drivers during different speeds of the train. From Myrtek et al., 1994, modified. Reproduced with permission (see Figure 26).

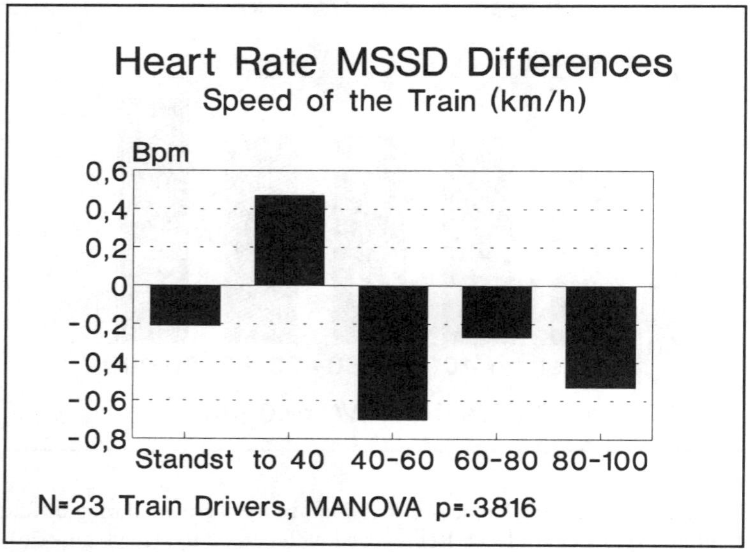

Figure 35. Heart rate variability MSSD (differences to baseline) in train drivers during different speeds of the train. From Myrtek et al., 1994, modified. Reproduced with permission (see Figure 26).

AHR showed no significant differences between the speed categories (see Figure 34). The relatively highest emotional impact was seen in "standstill" presumably caused by the interaction with other personal at the station. Heart rate variability, too, revealed no significant differences (see Figure 35).

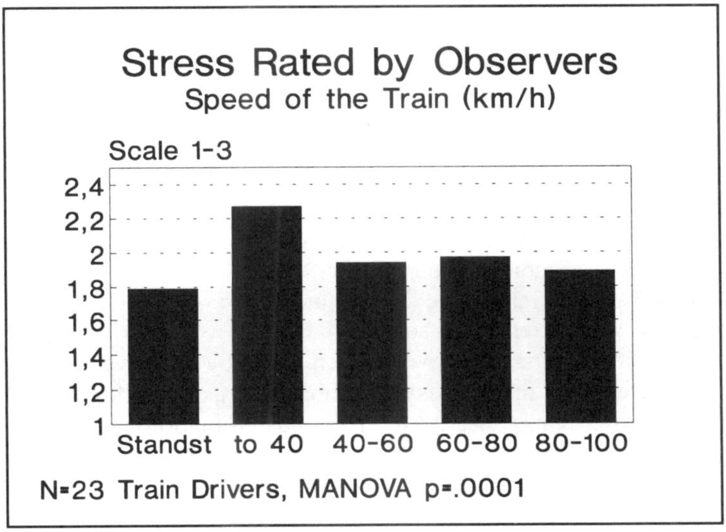

Figure 36. Stress ratings by the observers during different speeds of the train. From Myrtek et al., 1994. Reproduced with permission (see Figure 26).

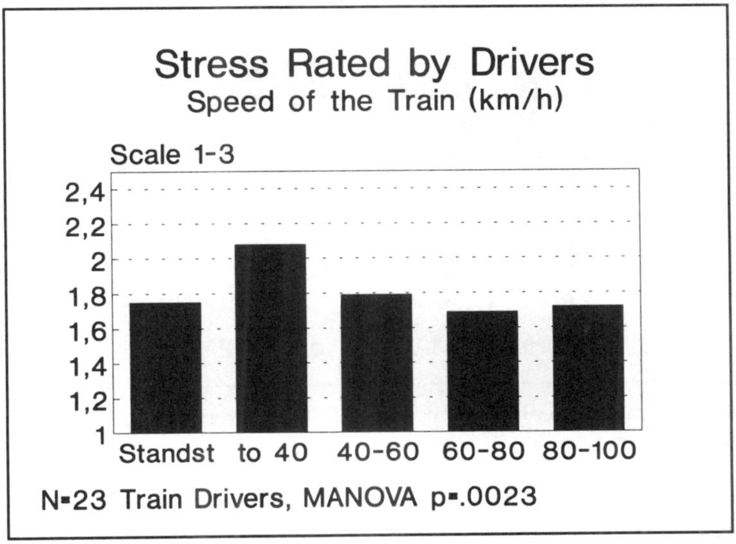

Figure 37. Stress ratings by the train drivers during different speeds of the train. From Myrtek et al., 1994. Reproduced with permission (see Figure 26).

Not in line with the foregoing results are the stress ratings made by the observers (see Figure 36). Here, "speeds up to 40 km/h" are rated as being stressful. Compared to this category all other speeds were rated as less stressful (p values .006 to $p < .001$). This corresponds rather well to the ratings made by the drivers themselves (see Figure 37; p values .001 to $p < .001$). However, there is again no correspondence with the physiological variables.

6.1.2 Work load in bus drivers

Thirteen bus drivers with a mean age of 46.0 years were accompanied in the bus by two trained observers. Actual work was characterized by the following categories:

- Number of braking actions for every minute with the categories "zero," "one," "two," and "three or more" actions.
- Stress of the situation rated for every minute by the observers: 3-step rating scale (no stress, moderate stress, high stress).
- Stress of the situation rated for every five minutes by the drivers themselves.

Heart rate increased with the increasing number of braking actions (see Figure 38). Compared to "zero braking," heart rate of the other situations was higher (p values .065 to $p = .001$).

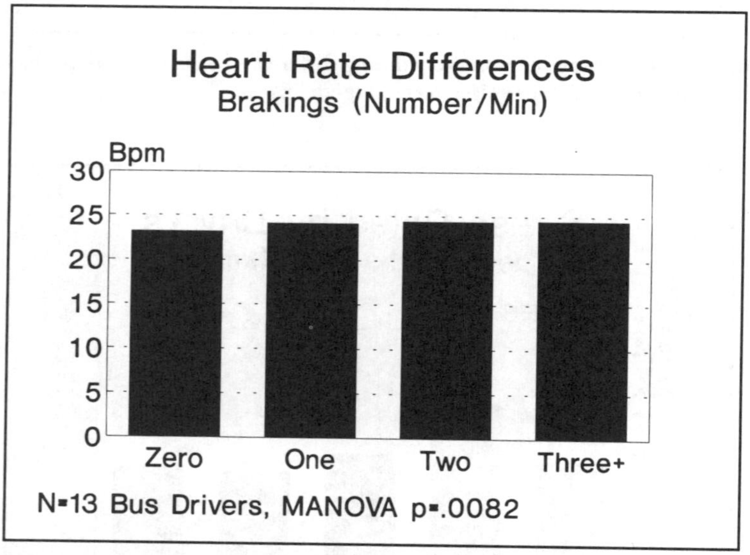

Figure 38. Heart rate (differences to baseline) in bus drivers during different numbers of braking actions per minute.

The increase in heart rate obviously was caused by the heightened physical activity (see Figure 39). Physical activity during minutes with braking actions was higher than during minutes without actions (p values .083 to $p = .009$).

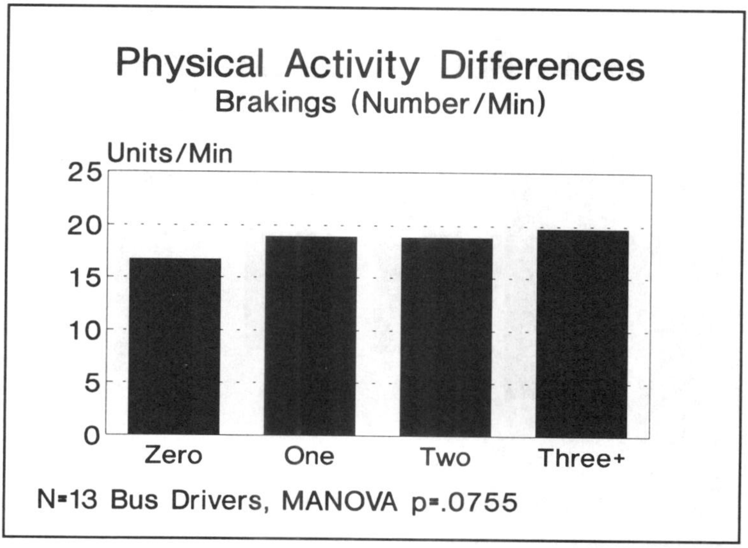

Figure 39. Physical activity (differences to baseline) in bus drivers during different numbers of braking actions per minute.

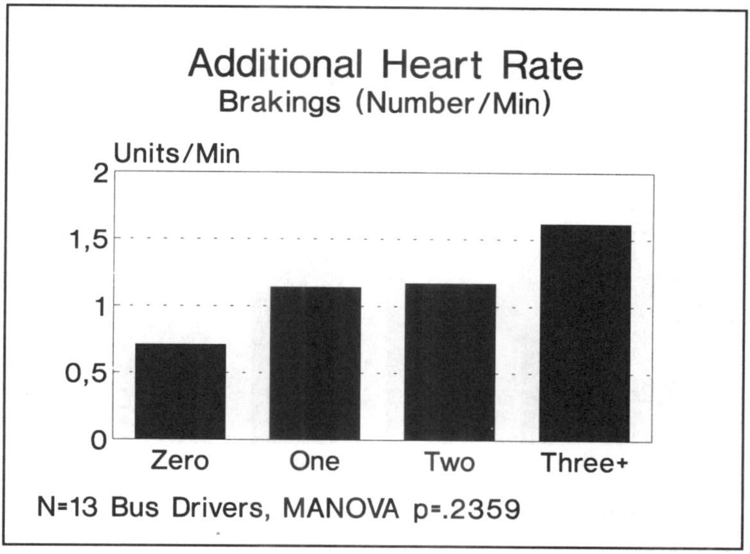

Figure 40. Additional heart rate in bus drivers during different numbers of braking actions per minute.

AHR also showed increasing figures (see Figure 40) but MANOVA was not significant, probably due to the relatively small sample size. In the bus drivers, too, heart rate variability (see Figure 41) was not significant.

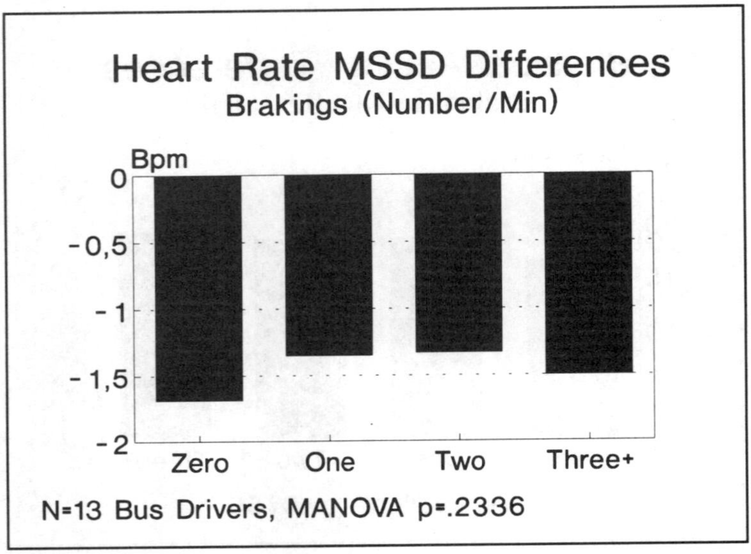

Figure 41. Heart rate variability MSSD (differences to baseline) in bus drivers during different numbers of braking actions per minute.

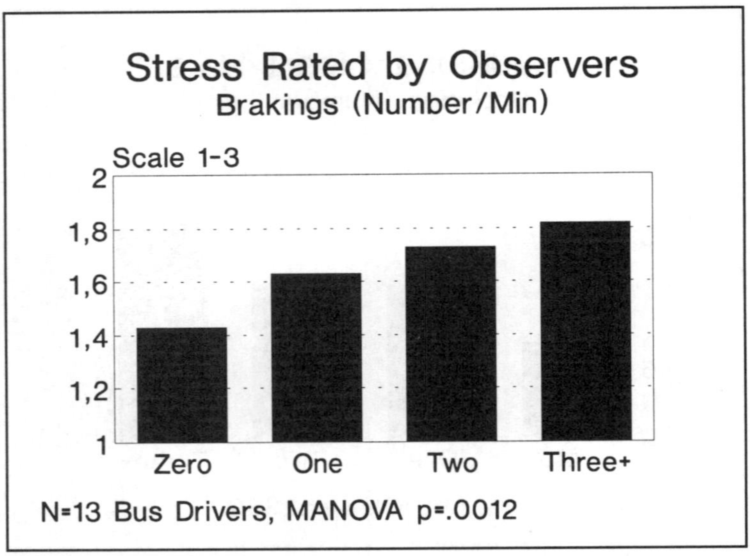

Figure 42. Stress ratings by the observers during different numbers of braking actions per minute.

Stress ratings made by the observers (see Figure 42) were in accordance with the physiological parameters. Apart from the stress ratings with "two" and "three or more" braking actions which did not differ, all other comparisons between the ratings were highly significant (p values .008 to $p < .001$) Ratings made by the bus drivers themselves showed no significant differences (see Figure 43).

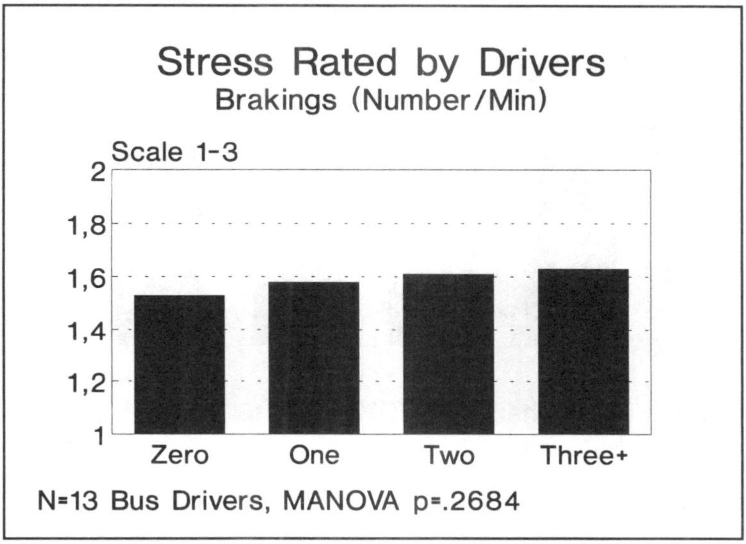

Figure 43. Stress ratings by the bus drivers during different numbers of braking actions per minute.

6.1.3 Work load in dispatchers

Thirteen dispatchers with a mean age of 46.5 years were observed by two observers in the signal tower. The dispatchers are responsible for the traffic into and out of the station. Similar to the train and bus drivers, their work was characterized by the following categories:

- Number of trains in the station for every minute with the categories "one to two," "three to four," "five to six," and "seven or more" trains in the station.
- Stress of the situation rated for every minute by the observers: 3-step rating scale (no stress, moderate stress, high stress).
- Stress of the situation rated for every five minutes by the drivers themselves.

Heart rate increased with the increasing number of trains for which dispatchers were responsible (see Figure 44). The differences between all heart rates were significant (p values .024 to $p < .001$). These heart rate increases were only partly due to more physical activity (see Figure 45).

Physical activity was highest when "five to six trains" were in the station. Comparisons with the other situations showed significant differences (p values .030 to $p = .002$). AHR was not significant, indicating no different emotional arousal for the differing numbers of trains in the station (see Figure 46). No significant differences for heart rate variability (see Figure 47) were observed.

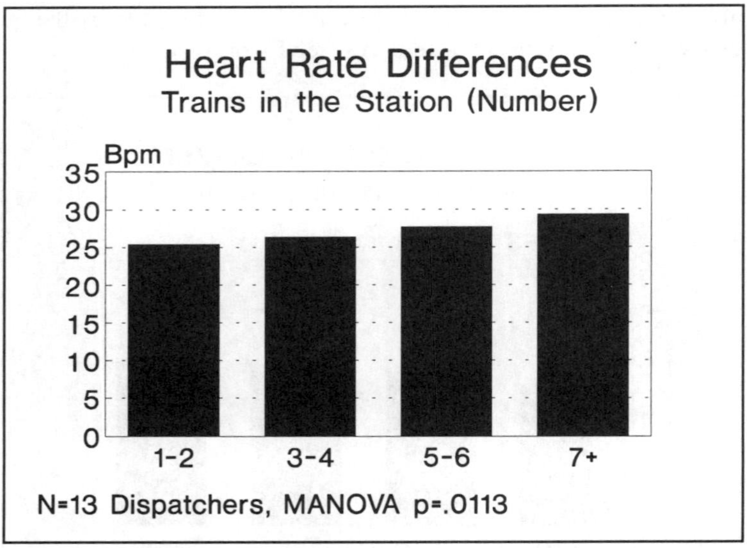

Figure 44. Heart rate (differences to baseline) in dispatchers during different numbers of trains in the station.

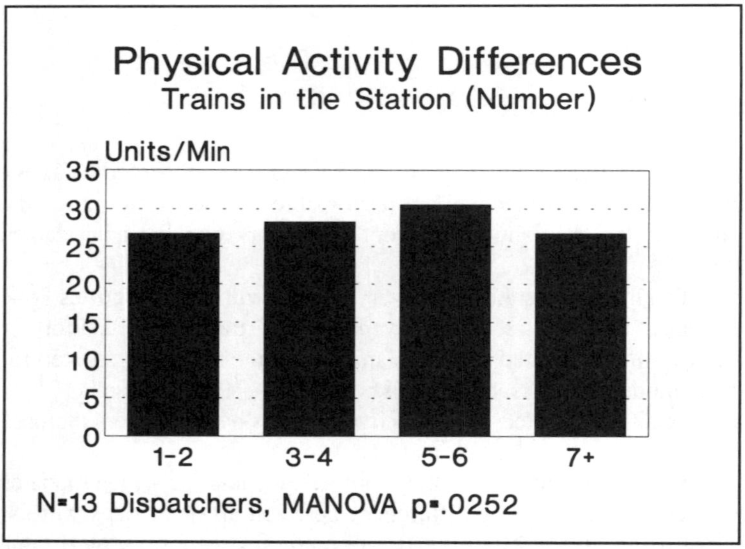

Figure 45. Physical activity (differences to baseline) in dispatchers during different numbers of trains in the station.

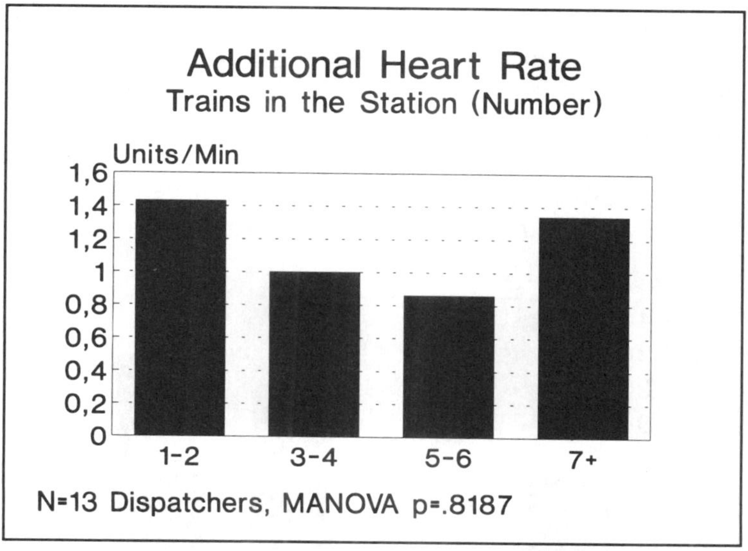

Figure 46. Additional heart rate in dispatchers during different numbers of trains in the station.

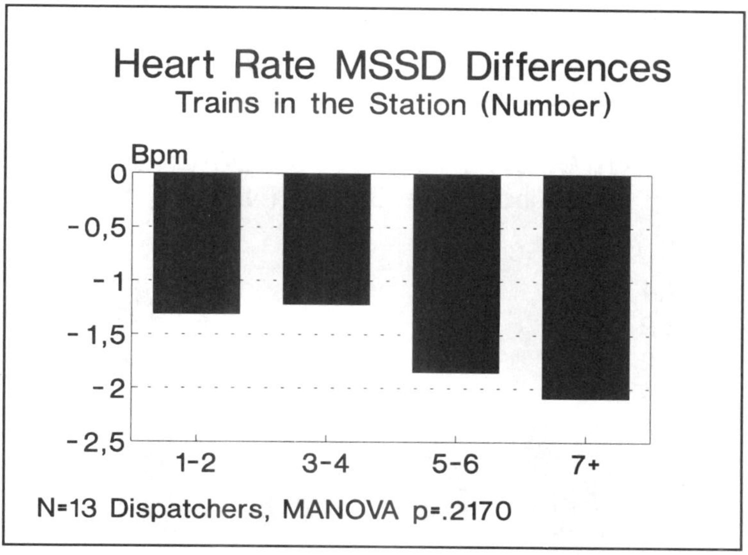

Figure 47. Heart rate variability MSSD (differences to baseline) in dispatchers during different numbers of trains in the station.

However, the stress ratings made by the observers were highly significantly different for the situations (see Figure 48; all p values < .001), with the exception of the comparison between "five to six" and "seven or more" trains (p = .058). Stress ratings made by the dispatchers themselves also showed a linear increase with the number of trains (see Figure 49). All comparisons between the differing categories were significant (p values .045 to $p < .001$).

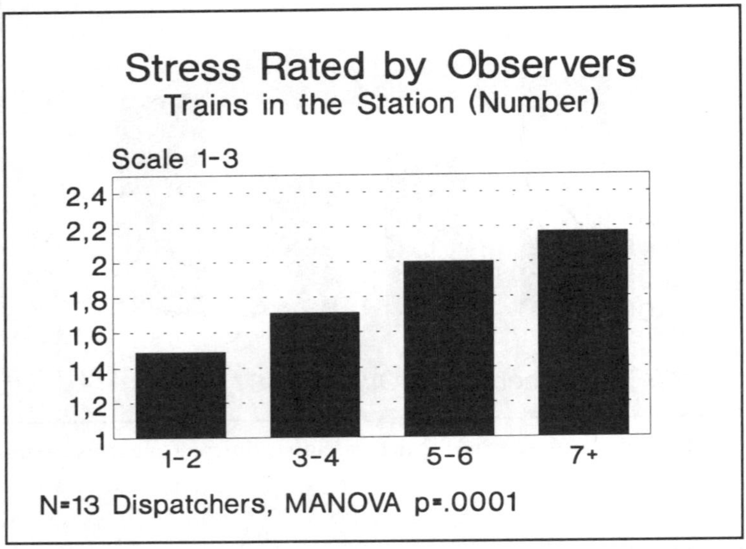

Figure 48. Stress ratings by the observers during different numbers of trains in the station.

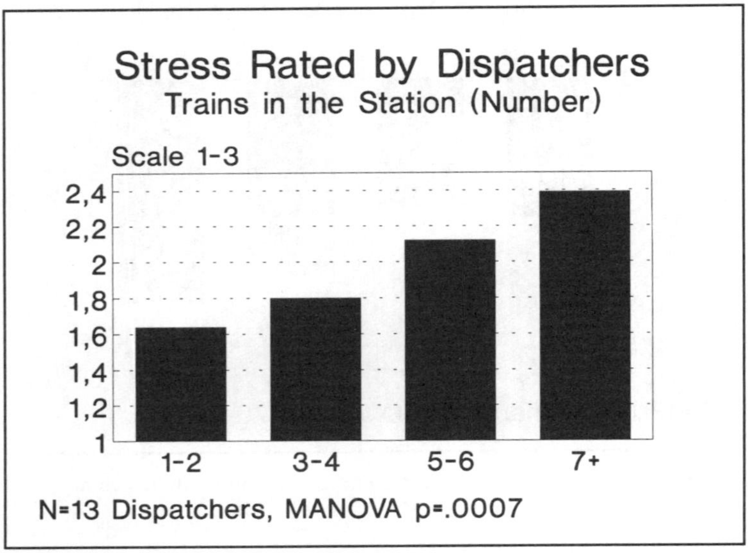

Figure 49. Stress ratings by the dispatchers during different numbers of trains in the station.

6.2 Work load in white and blue collar workers

The sample consisted of 106 blue and white collar workers of a big industrial plant producing plastics (Myrtek, Fichtler, Strittmatter, & Brügner, 1999; sample 17). Out of this sample, seven subjects were recorded only during leisure time and 13 subjects worked revolving shift, leaving 86 subjects with normal shift for the present analyses. Fifty-seven subjects were white collar workers (engineers, technologists, employees in the administration; mean age 51.2 years) and 29 blue collar workers (operators, craftsman; mean age 50.5 years). Complete records including the whole working time were obtained for 45 white and 22 blue collar workers. MANOVAs were used in a two-factorial design with the factors "working hours" (8.00 to 16.00 h) and "employees" (white vs. blue collar).

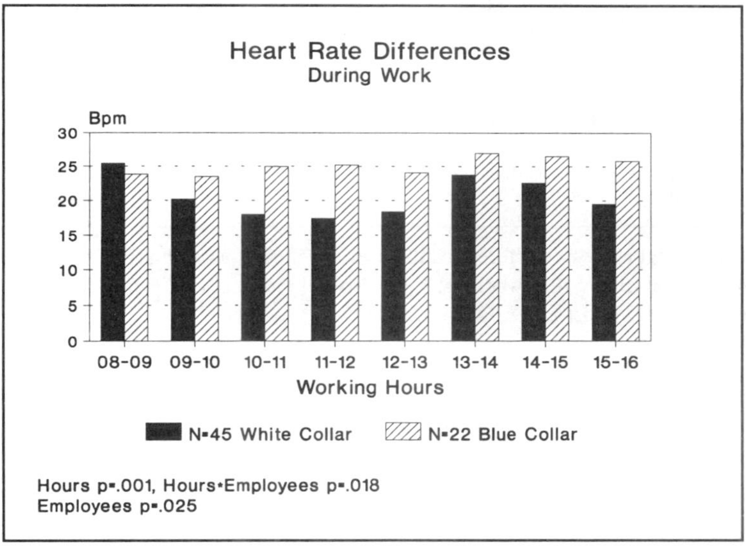

Figure 50. Heart rate (differences to baseline) during working time from 8.00 to 16.00 h among white and blue collar workers. From Myrtek et al., 1999. Reproduced with permission. Copyright 1999 by Elsevier, Oxford.

Heart rate (see Figure 50) was higher for blue than for white collar workers, obviously caused by the higher physical activity of the former group (see Figure 51). The working hours showed a significant main effect for both heart rate and physical activity. Physical activity was lowest between 12.00 and 13.00 h, presumably caused by the lunch break. This is also mirrored by heart rate. Both groups showed a differential trend in time, indicated by the significant interactions. However, we cannot interpret this trend because no task specific questions were posed. AHR (see Figure 52) revealed no significant difference between the groups but varied between the working hours. A small peak can be observed between 12.00 and 13.00 h. This is possibly due to the lunch break during which the employees had contact with other employees. Heart rate variability showed no significant main effects or interactions (see Figure 53).

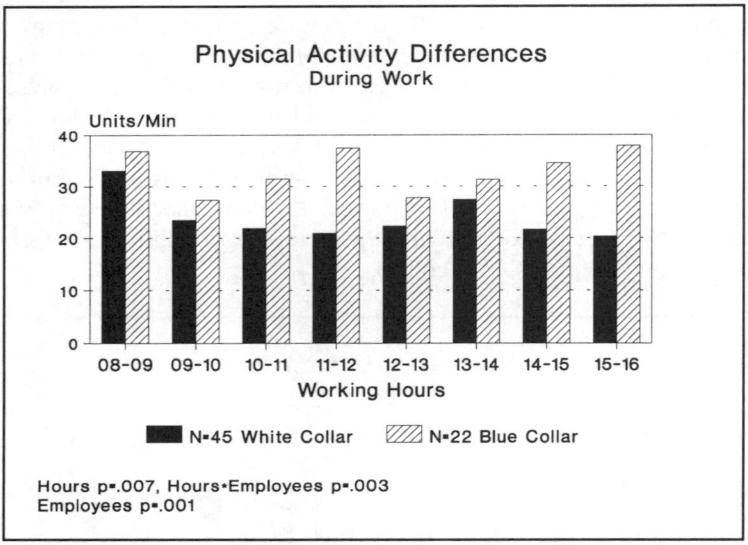

Figure 51. Physical activity (differences to baseline) during working time from 8.00 to 16.00 h among white and blue collar workers. From Myrtek et al., 1999. Reproduced with permission. Copyright 1999 by Elsevier, Oxford.

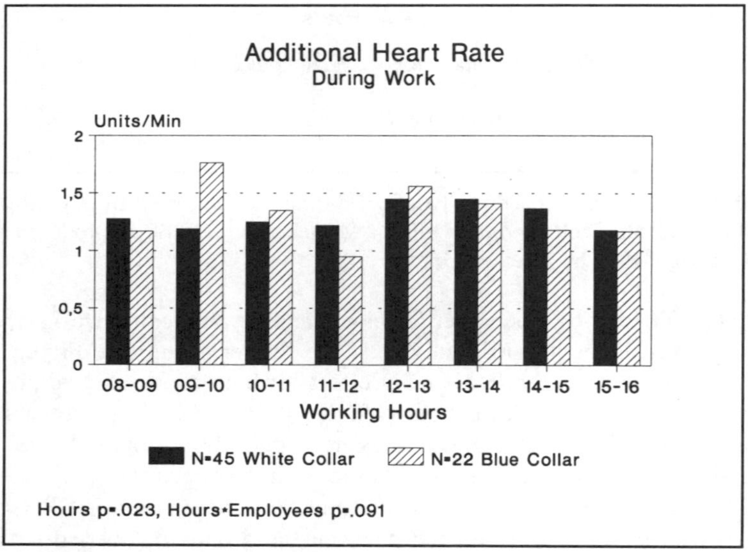

Figure 52. Additional heart rate during working time from 8.00 to 16.00 h among white and blue collar workers. From Myrtek et al., 1999. Reproduced with permission. Copyright 1999 by Elsevier, Oxford.

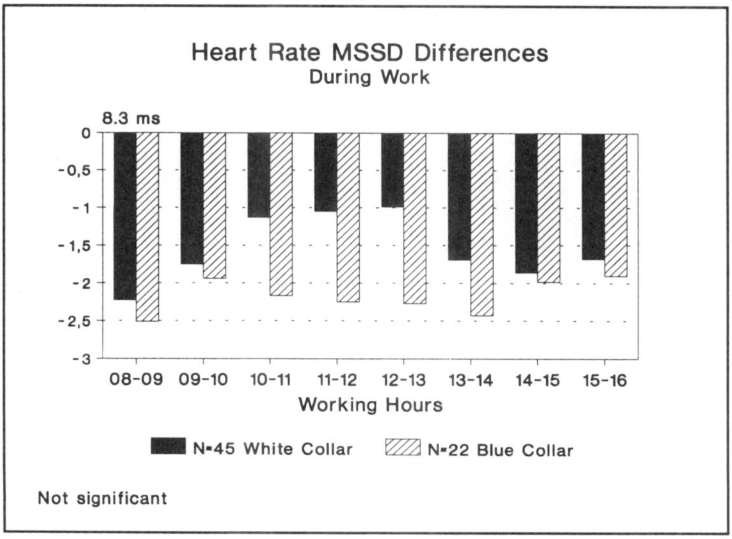

Figure 53. Heart rate variability MSSD (differences to baseline) during working time from 8.00 to 16.00 h among white and blue collar workers. From Myrtek et al., 1999. Reproduced with permission. Copyright 1999 by Elsevier, Oxford.

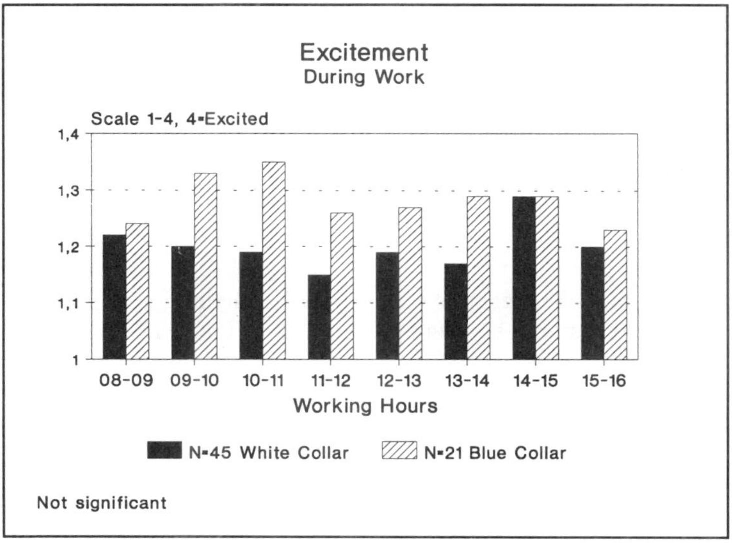

Figure 54. Excitement during working time from 8.00 to 16.00 h among white and blue collar workers. From Myrtek et al., 1999. Reproduced with permission. Copyright 1999 by Elsevier, Oxford.

The self-ratings of excitement and enjoyment showed no significant main effects for working hours or for groups (see Figures 54 and 55). Only a significant interaction for enjoyment was observed.

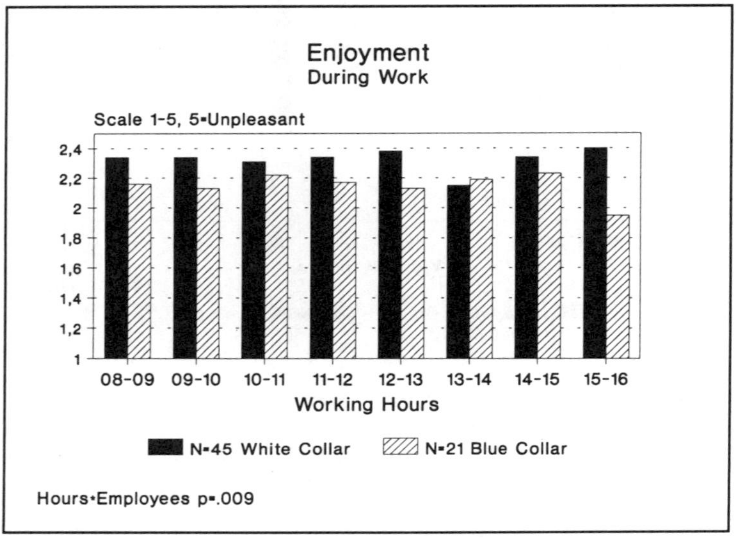

Figure 55. Enjoyment during working time from 8.00 to 16.00 h among white and blue collar workers. From Myrtek et al., 1999. Reproduced with permission. Copyright 1999 by Elsevier, Oxford.

6.3 Work load in university students

6.3.1 First study

In a first study, 50 female (mean age 23.4 years; sample 8) and 50 male students (mean age 23.7 years; sample 11) were examined with the FMS during everyday life (Myrtek, Hilgenberg, Brügner, & Müller, 1997). The physiological and psychological parameters were assessed with our device both while at the university and at home. On the day of ambulatory monitoring, all male students attended the university but only 40 female students, thus reducing the sample to $N = 90$. Our hypothesis was that time spent at the university as compared to staying at home will show generally higher physiological reactivity.

Comparisons between study-related and leisure activities revealed no differences in physical activity, but heart rate, indicating total work load, was higher while studying, especially for men (see Figures 56 and 57). AHR was higher at the university than at home (see Figure 58) and female students showed more AHR than male students.

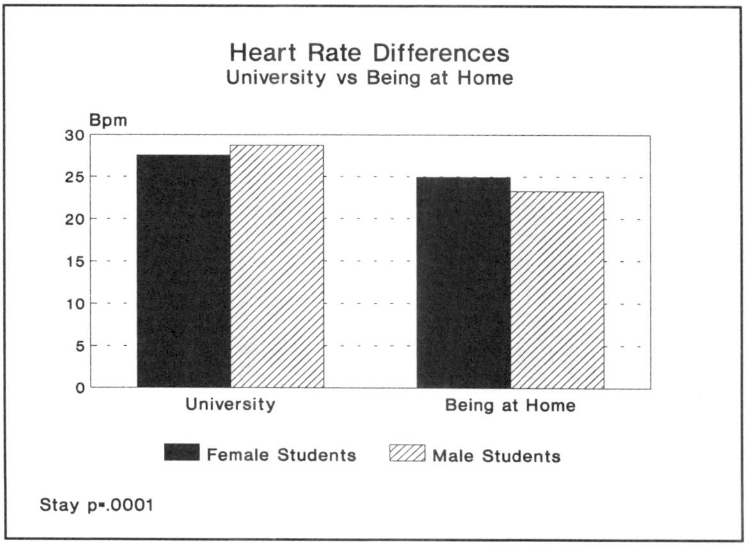

Figure 56. Heart rate (differences to baseline) staying at the university or at home in female and male students. From Myrtek et al., 1997, modified. Reproduced with permission. Copyright 1997 by the Federation of European Psychophysiology Societies.

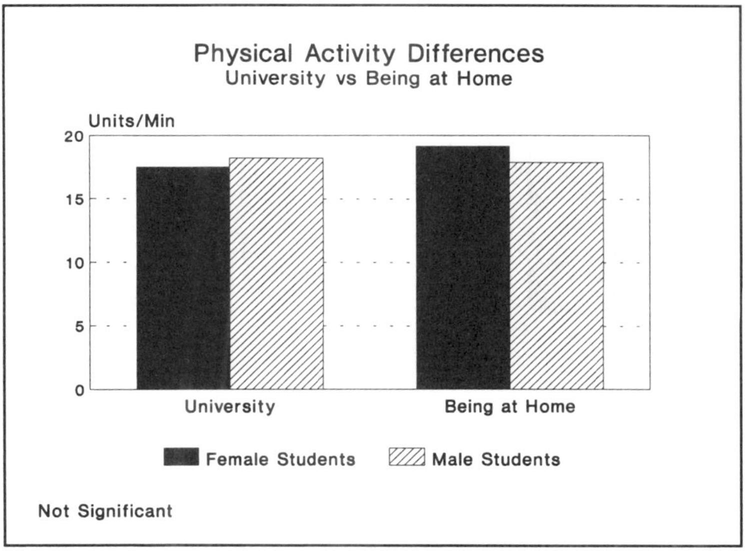

Figure 57. Physical activity (differences to baseline) staying at the university or at home in female and male students. From Myrtek et al., 1997, modified. Reproduced with permission. Copyright 1997 by the Federation of European Psychophysiology Societies.

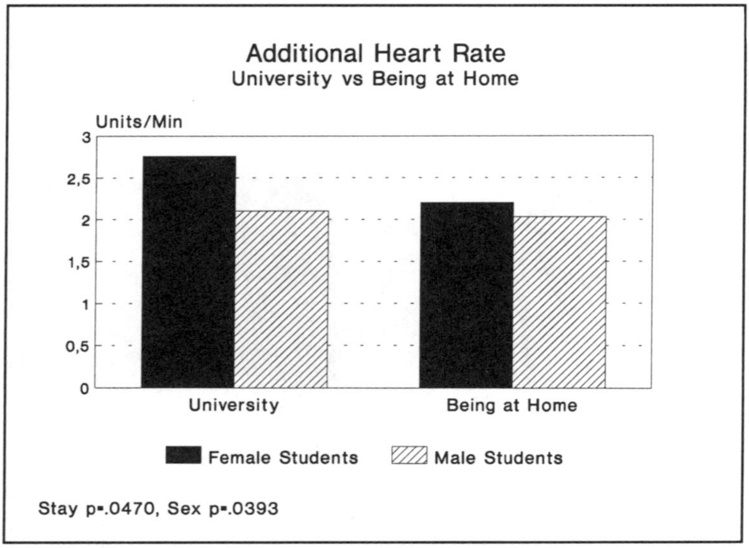

Figure 58. Additional heart rate staying at the university or at home in female and male students. From Myrtek et al., 1997, modified. Reproduced with permission. Copyright 1997 by the Federation of European Psychophysiology Societies.

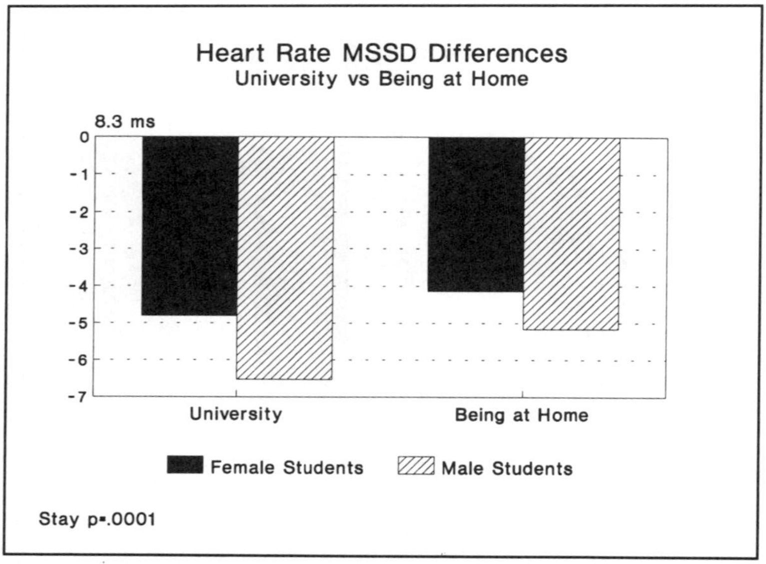

Figure 59. Heart rate variability MSSD (differences to baseline) staying at the university or at home in female and male students. From Myrtek et al., 1997, modified. Reproduced with permission. Copyright 1997 by the Federation of European Psychophysiology Societies.

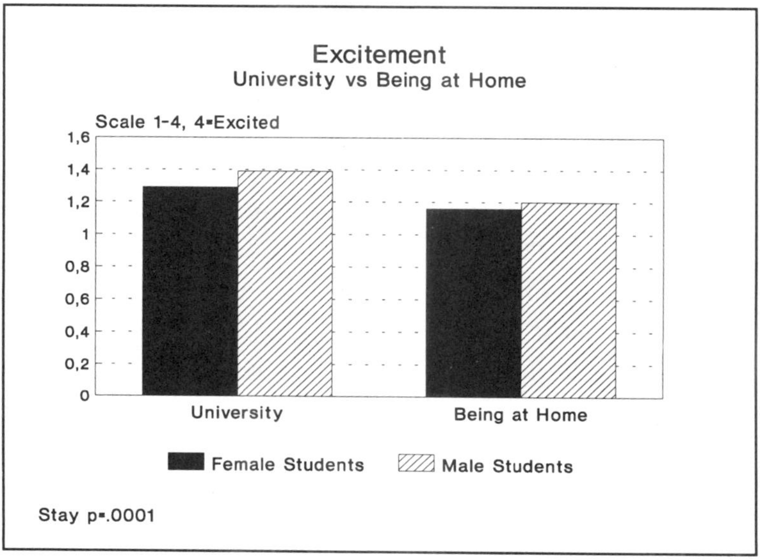

Figure 60. Excitement staying at the university or at home in female and male students. From Myrtek et al., 1997, modified. Reproduced with permission. Copyright 1997 by the Federation of European Psychophysiology Societies.

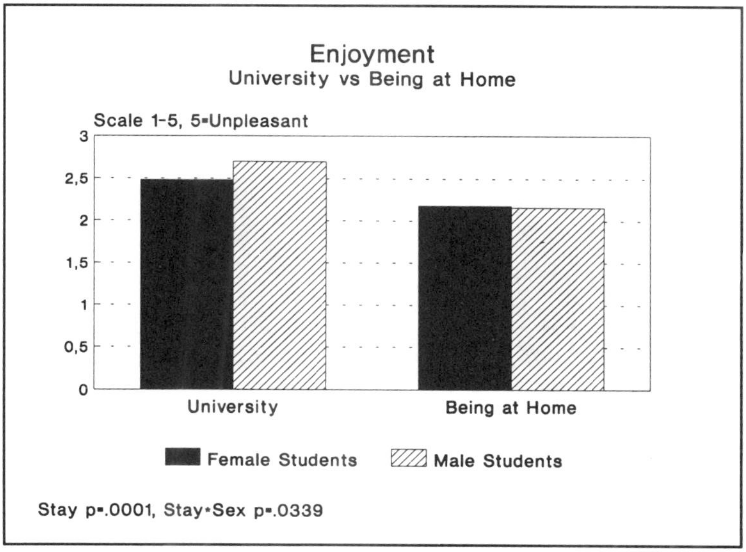

Figure 61. Enjoyment staying at the university or at home in female and male students. From Myrtek et al., 1997, modified. Reproduced with permission. Copyright 1997 by the Federation of European Psychophysiology Societies.

Heart rate variability MSSD (see Figure 59) revealed higher responses at the university, thus supporting the notion that heart rate variability might be an indicator of mental work load. After controlling for heart rate, however, the difference between university and home was no longer significant (p = .443).

Students generally rated activities at home as less exciting (see Figure 60) and more enjoyable (see Figure 61) than their studies. The interaction for enjoyment denotes that male as compared to female students enjoyed being at the university even less, with no difference when at home.

6.3.2 Replication study

In the replication study, 50 female (mean age 22.3 years; sample 12) and 50 male students (mean age 23.3 years; sample 13) were examined in the same way as in the first study. On the day of ambulatory monitoring, all female students attended the university but only 47 male students, thus reducing the sample to $N = 97$.

Because physical activity in these samples was significantly higher at home than at the university (see Figure 63), the heart rate difference (see Figure 62) between being at the university and being at home was obscured. After controlling for physical activity, the heart rate difference between university and home was significant (p = .017), thus confirming the result of the first study.

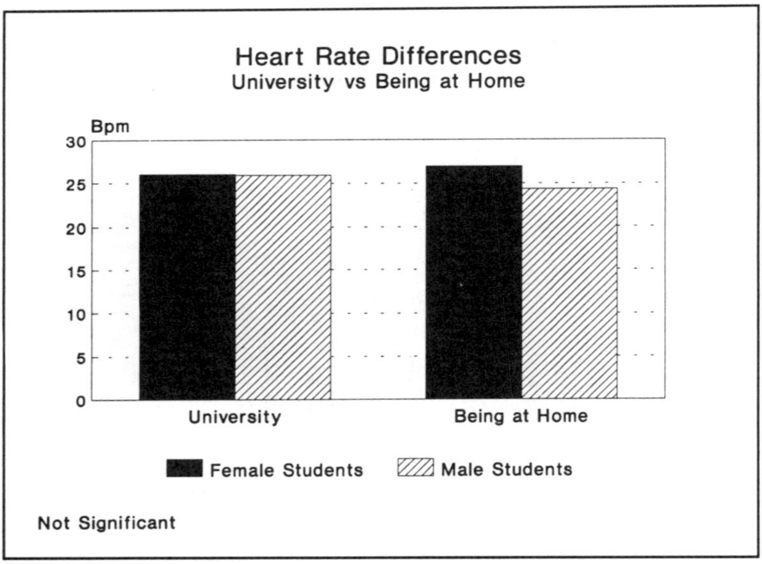

Figure 62. Heart rate (differences to baseline) staying at the university or at home in female and male students.

AHR (see Figure 64) was not different between staying at the university and staying at home. As in the first study, heart rate variability MSSD (see Figure 65) showed higher responses at the university. After controlling for heart rate, the difference between university and home was no longer significant ($p = .262$).

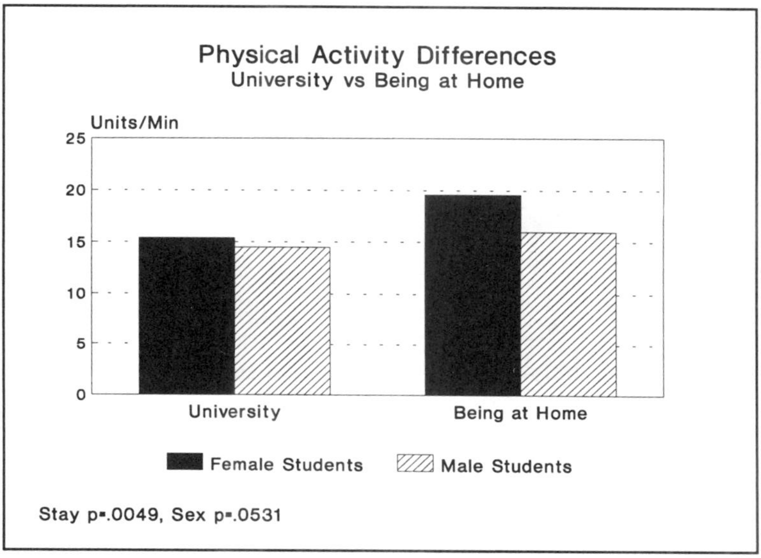

Figure 63. Physical activity (differences to baseline) staying at the university or at home in female and male students.

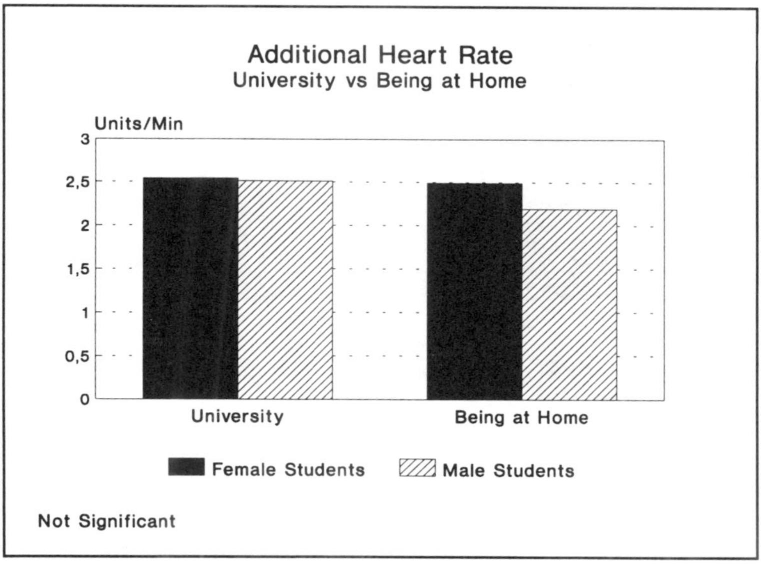

Figure 64. Additional heart rate staying at the university or at home in female and male students.

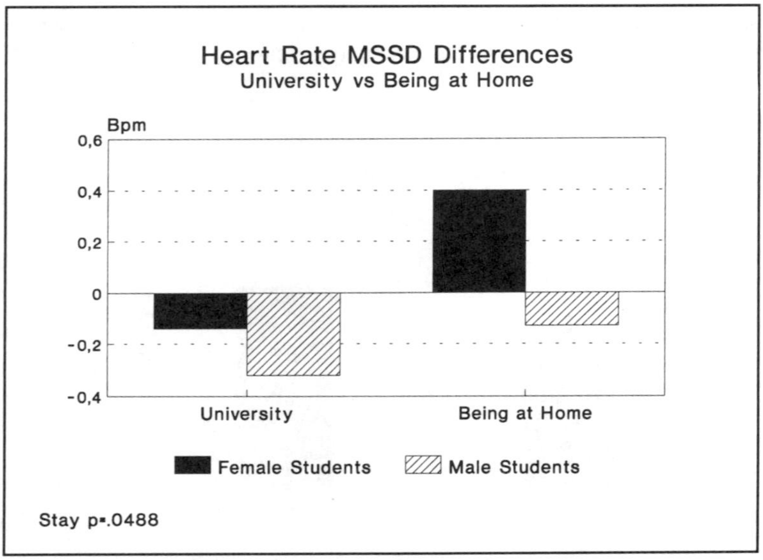

Figure 65. Heart rate variability MSSD (differences to baseline) staying at the university or at home in female and male students.

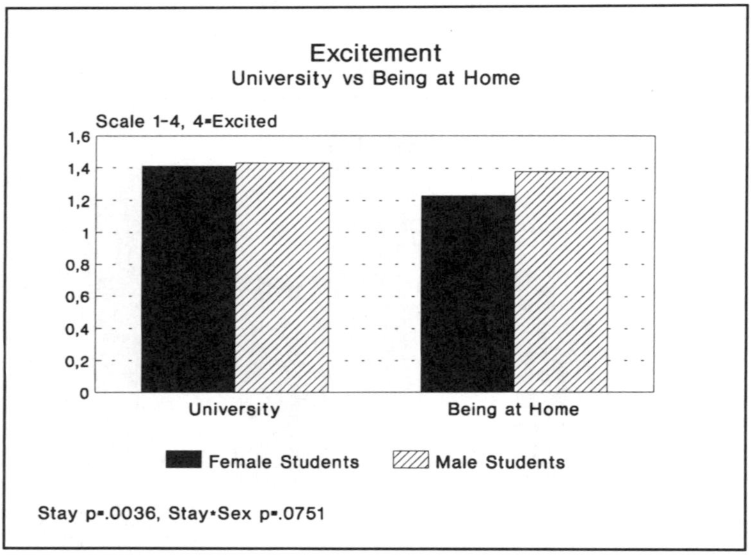

Figure 66. Excitement staying at the university or at home in female and male students.

Similar to the first study, students rated activities at home as less exciting (see Figure 66) and more enjoyable (see Figure 67) than their studies. The interaction for excitement means that male students were more excited in both situations, whereas female students showed less excitement when they were at home.

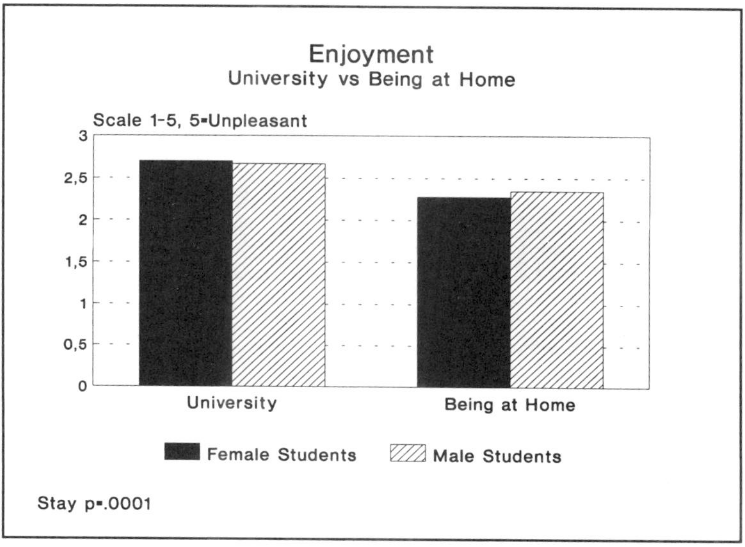

Figure 67. Enjoyment staying at the university or at home in female and male students.

6.4 Work load in schoolboys

Hundred schoolboys in the 5th and 6th grades (mean age 11.1 years; sample 6) and 100 schoolboys in the 9th and 10th grades (mean age 15.4 years; sample 7) were monitored with the FMS on a normal school day (Monday to Friday). Monitoring began at school on the first day and lasted till the second day while boys were at school. It was therefore possible to record lessons in the same subject twice on different days in several boys. We were interested in whether the work load in lessons with a classroom test or lessons during which the results of these tests were announced would be different than in normal lessons in the same subject in which no tests were given. Of the younger boys, 29 had both lessons and 45 of the older boys were in both situations on the day of monitoring.

Heart rate (see Figure 68) was higher during lessons with classroom tests as compared to normal lessons. However, physical activity (see Figure 69) was also marginally higher during the classroom tests. Therefore, heart rate was controlled for physical activity which reduced the level of significance to $p = .053$. Generally, heart rate reactivity was higher in older than in younger boys. AHR (see Figure 70) and heart rate variability (see Figure 71) showed no significant differences for classroom tests compared to normal lessons.

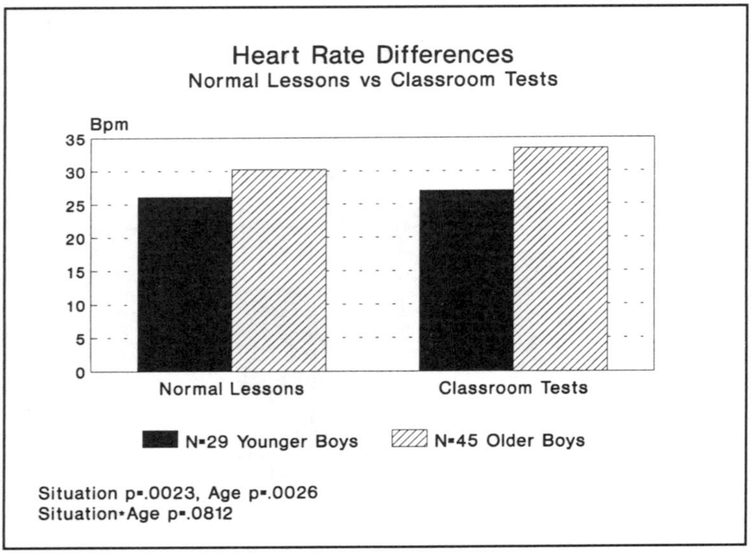

Figure 68. Heart rate (differences to baseline) during normal lessons versus classroom tests in schoolboys. From Myrtek & Scharff, 2000, modified. Reproduced with permission. Copyright 2000 by Huber, Bern.

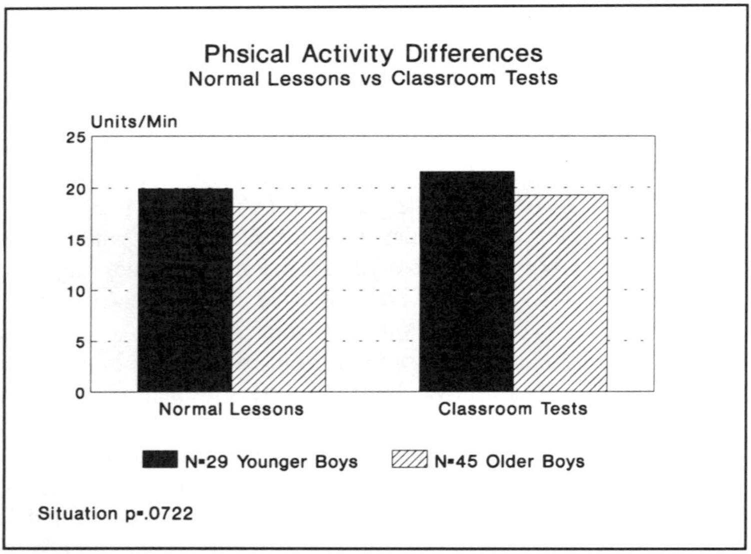

Figure 69. Physical activity (differences to baseline) during normal lessons versus classroom tests in schoolboys.

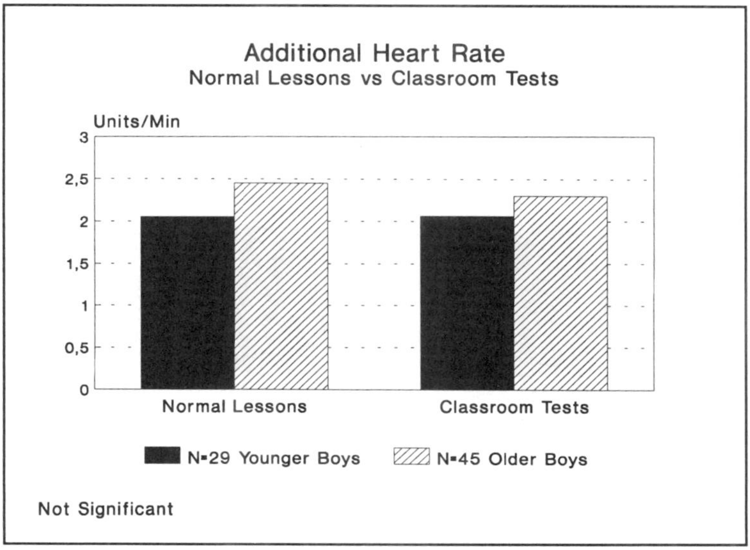

Figure 70. Additional heart rate during normal lessons versus classroom tests in schoolboys. From Myrtek & Scharff, 2000, modified. Reproduced with permission. Copyright 2000 by Huber, Bern.

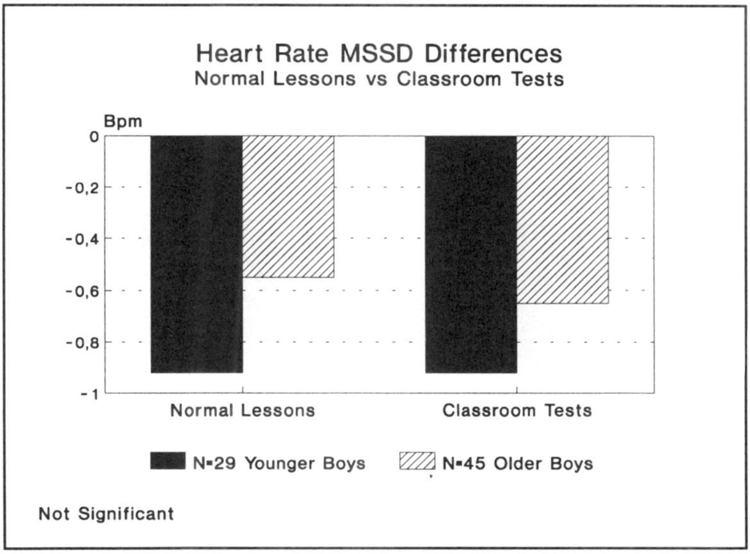

Figure 71. Heart rate variability MSSD (differences to baseline) during normal lessons versus classroom tests in schoolboys.

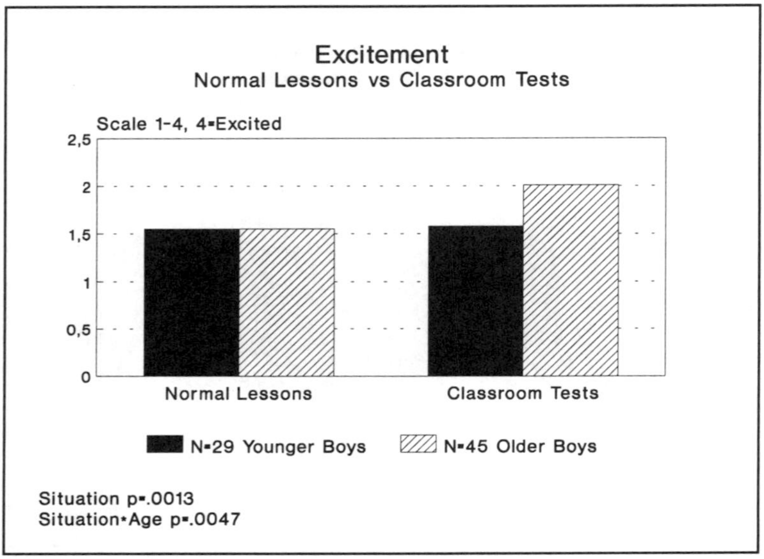

Figure 72. Excitement during normal lessons versus classroom tests in schoolboys. From Myrtek & Scharff, 2000, modified. Reproduced with permission. Copyright 2000 by Huber, Bern.

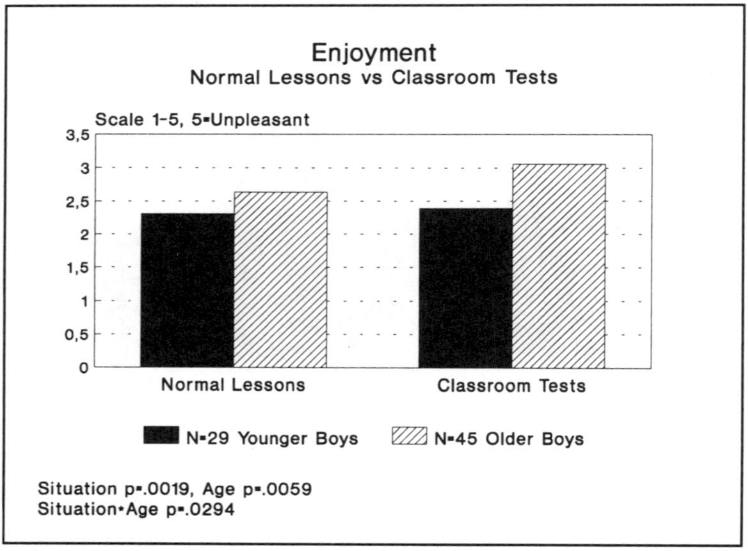

Figure 73. Enjoyment during normal lessons versus classroom tests in schoolboys. From Myrtek & Scharff, 2000, modified. Reproduced with permission. Copyright 2000 by Huber, Bern.

Striking differences, however, were observed for excitement (see Figure 72) and enjoyment (see Figure 73). Classroom tests were rated to be more exciting and less enjoyable than normal lessons with the same subject. The older boys rated school time to be less enjoyable than did the younger boys. The significant interaction situation * age denotes that the older boys were still more excited and less enjoyed during the classroom test than the younger boys.

6.5 Discussion

In this Chapter the possibility to examine with the FMS the work load of different occupational groups was demonstrated. Since the work performed by man is increasingly characterized by low physical but high emotional and mental work load, it is important to differentiate the work load components within a specific task. Stress ratings made by the working subject or by an observer are important, too, although these are not necessarily valid indicators of the strain imposed on the subject. Frauendorf and Kobryn (1975) published guidelines for the evaluation of physical labor. According to these guidelines, heart rate increases above baseline of up to 20 bpm are regarded as characteristic of light, 20 to 30 bpm middle heavy, 30 to 40 bpm heavy, and above 40 bpm of very heavy physical labor.

6.5.1 Train drivers, bus drivers, and dispatchers

These occupational groups showed heart rate increases between 20 and 30 bpm. According to the guidelines cited above, their physical work might be characterized as light to middle heavy.

In train drivers, heart rate as the component of total workload was lowest during "moving" as compared to other modes of driving such as "start," "braking to halt," and "standstill." The driving modes "start" and "braking to halt" are examples of the emotional work load component (AHR). Driving into the station and leaving the station bears a heightened risk for accidents with passengers standing near the track. This may be the reason for the increase in this work load component. Important is the fact that certain situations with high work load as indicated by the physiological variables, e.g., "start," were not adequately rated, be it by the observers or the drivers. This finding coincides with that of Benzer, Niebergall, Posch, and Flora (1991) in their study with doctors on emergency calls. This means that the analysis of work load cannot be done adequately on the basis of subjective or observer derived stress ratings alone. No significant differences were observed for heart rate variability, the commonly used indicator of mental work load.

The different train speeds revealed no significant differences for heart rate, AHR, and heart rate variability. Physical activity increased spuriously due to the vibrations of the engine and not due to physical activity. Therefore, we have to conclude that increasing speeds up to 100 km/h are not associated with an increasing work load.

Higher speeds up to 200 km/h even showed a monotony effect with a decrease in heart rate. Contrary to these findings, stress rated by the observers and by the drivers differentiated the train speeds with higher stress during speeds up to 40 km/h.

The bus drivers revealed increasing heart rate with increasing number of times they engaged the brakes. This increase was primarily caused by the increasing physical activity during braking. AHR also showed an increase with more braking but was statistically not significant. Again heart rate variability revealed no differences between the number of "brakings." The observer rated more stress with more "brakings" but the ratings made by the drivers were not different.

Total work load of the dispatchers as indicated by heart rate was dependent on the number of trains dispatchers had to manage at the same time. This was partly due to the heightened physical activity. AHR and heart rate variability, however, revealed no significant differences. The ratings both by the observers and the dispatchers themselves were in line with the total work load.

6.5.2 White and blue collar workers

As was expected, responses for heart rate and physical activity during work were higher for blue collar than for white collar workers, indicating more total work load and physical work load for the former group. Total heart rate response during working hours was 26 bpm for the blue collar and 21 bpm for the white collar workers. However, raw heart rate scores during work were nearly the same for both groups, 82 bpm for blue and 81 bpm for white collar workers. Therefore, basal heart rate was about four bpm higher for the white collar group. Obviously, the blue collar workers were physically fitter than the white collar workers. This result underlines the necessity for an adequate baseline to evaluate work load. As already stated for the train drivers, bus drivers, and dispatchers, physical work load was light to middle heavy even for the industrial blue collar workers.

Heart rate and physical activity showed significant trends during the working hours from 8.00 h to 16.00 h, but it was not possible to interpret these trends in detail because work specific activities were not assessed. The relatively low physical activity at 12.00 h to 13.00 h obviously indicated lunch break. This interpretation was supported by the higher AHR at this time which was presumably due to social contacts with other employees. As stated in Chapter 3.4.3.5, social contacts with other persons can notably raise AHR, especially during contact with persons with whom subjects are not well acquainted. During the last half of the working shift, heart rate showed a tendency to increase, which might be due to increasing fatigue or circadian variation.

According to several authors (e.g., Nerell & Wahlund, 1981), white collar workers are subjected to higher mental work load, whereas blue collar workers are subjected to higher physical work load as shown by our results. However, no differences between blue and white collar workers were observed either for heart rate variability, indicating mental work load, or for AHR, indicating emotional work load. The notion that mental work load is higher in white collar workers derives from interviews and questionnaire data but not from physiological measurements at the workplace. In a questionnaire used in the present study, stress at work was rated significantly higher by the white collar than by the blue collar workers confirming this prejudice. The ratings of excitement and enjoyment during work, which are based on the mean of more than 20 feedbacks per subject, showed no differences between the groups. This is in line with the physiological findings but contradicts the stress rating in the questionnaire. An explanation might be seen in the so-called negative retrospection effect (Fahrenberg, Leonhart, & Foerster, 2002; Käppler & Rieder, 2001). This effect is based on the observation that subjects' stress ratings are significantly different during actual monitoring as compared to a retrospective evaluation after monitoring, the latter indicating higher stress. The retrospective ratings might be influenced by cognitive schemas more than the actual ratings during work. It may be that white collar workers are more acquainted with the stress concept than blue collar workers. We have already pointed out the important point of cognitive schemas in Chapters 4 and 5.

6.5.3 University students

Students often complain of stress while at the university (Campbell, Svenson, & Jarvis, 1992). Apart from studies designed to isolate the effects of acute psychological stress during examinations (Fuller, 1992; Sausen et al., 1992), no studies have investigated possible stress effects obtained during normal university life. We have examined this issue with the FMS in a first study with 50 female and 50 male students and tried to replicate the results in a second study with 50 female and 50 male students. Therefore, we can interpret the replicated results with high certainty.

Heart rate, controlled for physical activity, was higher at the university as compared to being at home in both sexes. Heart rate response at the university was above 25 bpm and in the same range as seen for the different occupational groups discussed above. Therefore, total work load is comparable to other employees. In the first study, AHR was also higher staying at the university, but this finding could not be replicated. Heart rate variability was significantly lower during the stay at the university in both studies. However, heart rate variability is not independent of heart rate itself as described in Chapter 3 (see Table 9). Multivariate analysis with heart rate as a covariate rendered both results insignificant. We may conclude, once more, that heart rate variability is a questionable parameter of mental work load.

Excitement was rated in both studies as higher at the university than at home. Similarly, enjoyment was greater at home than at university. In the first study, a significant interaction stay * sex was observed, whereby male students enjoyed university life still less than female students. But this result could not be replicated. The findings are indicators of mild, acute, subjective stress imposed on the students, and are consistent with those of Sausen et al. (1992).

6.5.4 Schoolboys

Classroom tests are rather unpopular among schoolboys. This is clearly demonstrated by the excitement ratings and enjoyment ratings recorded during the tests compared to normal lessons in the same subject. Interestingly, the ratings of the older boys revealed even more excitement and less enjoyment during the tests compared to the younger boys as indicated by the significant interactions situation * age. It may be concluded that such tests are more relevant for the older boys because their marks are important for later occupational decisions.

The relevance of classroom tests for the older boys is also mirrored by the heart rate responses with higher responses during the tests. Moreover, heart rate response was generally higher in older than in younger boys although physical activity was somewhat lower in the former group. This also indicates the higher importance of lessons in the older boys. AHR was numerically somewhat higher in the older boys but did not reach the level of significance. Again, heart rate variability showed no significant differences.

6.6 Summary

On a normal working day, 23 train drivers, 13 bus drivers, and 13 dispatchers were studied with the FMS. Two observers accompanied the subjects during work and rated the special work tasks for about two working hours. Observed stress of the situation was rated every minute by the observers and every five minute by the subjects themselves, respectively.

In the train drivers, mode of driving (start, moving, change of speed, coming to a halt, and standstill) and speed of the train (standstill, up to 40 km/h, 40 to 60 km/h, 60 to 80 km/h, and 80 to 100 km/h) was rated for every minute by the observers. In all groups physical activity was light to middle heavy with heart rate increases between 20 to 30 bpm above baseline. Total work load was lowest in train drivers during movement compared to the other modes of driving. AHR was especially high during start and braking to a halt. The explanation for this is seen in the heightened risk for accidents during these modes. However, these situations were not rated in the same way as indicated by the physiological variables be it by the observers or the drivers themselves. The different train speeds showed no significant work load differences.

The observers counted the number of braking actions per minute performed by bus drivers (zero, one, two, and three or more). Heart rate increased with the number of braking actions due to increasing physical activity. AHR also increased but was statistically not significant. Stress as rated by the observers increased also but the bus drivers' own stress ratings were not significant.

In the dispatchers, the number of trains in the station per minute (one to two, three to four, five to six, and seven or more) was rated by the observers. Heart rate increased with the number of trains which the dispatchers had to manage but this was partly due to the increasing physical activity. The subjective ratings both by the observers and the subjects were in line with the increase of total work load. Heart rate variability, the commonly regarded indicator of mental work load, was not significant in all groups.

In a second study with 45 white and 22 blue collar workers, work load during a normal shift was examined. Total work load and physical work load were higher in blue than in white collar workers. At 12.00 h to 13.00 h physical activity was lower and AHR was relatively higher compared to other working hours, presumably caused by the lunch break. Subjects' ratings of excitement and enjoyment were not significantly different between white and blue collar workers and also showed no main effect over the working day. Again, heart rate variability was not significant.

In two other studies, each with 100 female and male university students, staying at the university was compared to being at home. Heart rate, controlled for physical activity, was higher at the university in both studies and both sexes. Heart rate variability was lower at the university, but was no longer significant after control for heart rate. Excitement was rated as higher at the university compared to being at home in both studies and both sexes, whereas enjoyment was rated as higher at home.

In our last study, classroom tests were compared to normal lessons on the same subject in 29 11-year-old and 45 15-year-old schoolboys. Total work load as indicated by heart rate was higher during classroom tests. Generally, heart rate response was higher in older than in younger boys indicating the higher importance of lessons in older boys. AHR and heart rate variability were not significantly different. As could be expected, excitement was higher during the tests and enjoyment was lower. Significant interactions situation * age in both ratings revealed that the older boys were still more excited and experienced less enjoyment during the tests compared to the younger boys.

Chapter 7

Stress and strain during leisure time

Generally, work is seen to cause stress and its concomitant physiological strain responses. Leisure time, however, is looked upon as being relaxing and restful. Presumably, these views are grounded in the fact that work always has a certain compulsory element, whereas leisure time has not. Another reason for these views surely results from the fact that psychophysiological studies on work are rare and on leisure time practically nonexistent. With the FMS we have a suitable instrument to compare work with leisure time and to answer the question whether leisure time is really as restful as people believe.

7.1 Work versus leisure time in train drivers, bus drivers, and dispatchers

In Chapter 6 we examined 23 train drivers, 13 bus drivers, and 13 dispatchers (drawn from sample 16) during their working time. Using 23h monitoring, we can also take a look at their leisure time.

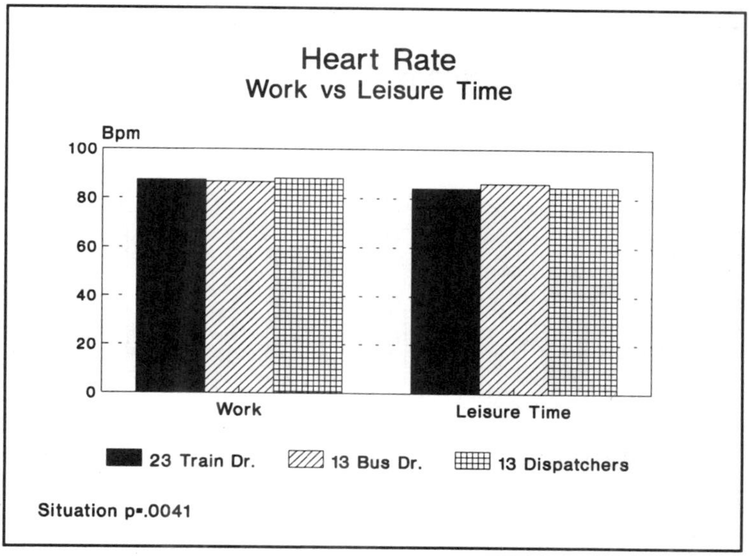

Figure 74. Heart rate in train drivers, bus drivers, and dispatchers during work and leisure time.

Heart rate (see Figure 74) was somewhat lower during leisure time in all groups with no group differences. The lower heart rate is due to the reduced physical activity during leisure time (see Figure 75).

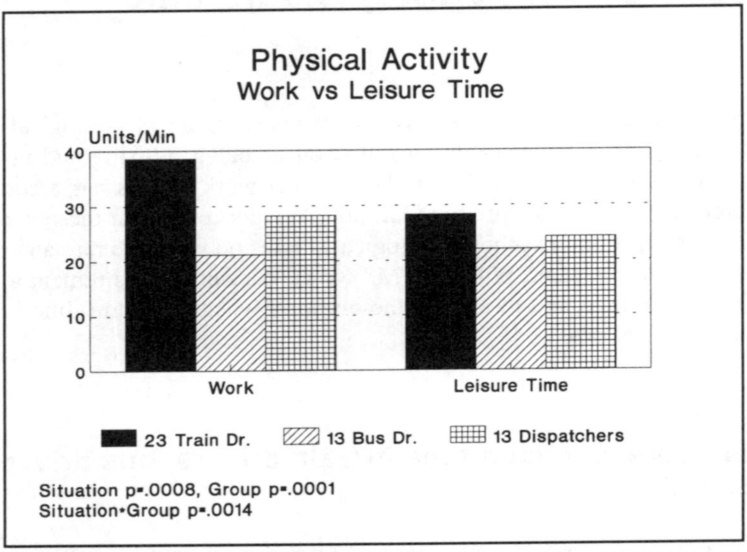

Figure 75. Physical activity in train drivers, bus drivers, and dispatchers during work and leisure time.

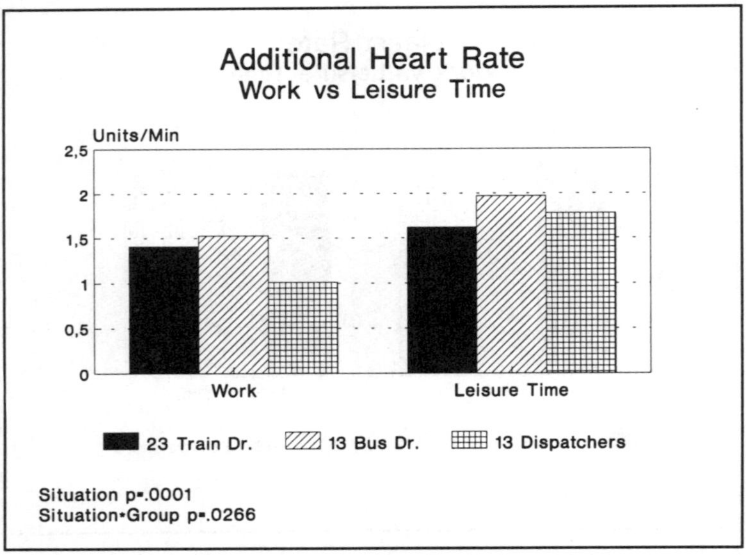

Figure 76. Additional heart rate in train drivers, bus drivers, and dispatchers during work and leisure time.

Physical activity is spuriously heightened in the train drivers at work. This is caused by the vibrations of the engine. Therefore, the significant group difference and interaction situation * group cannot be interpreted as genuine different physical activity of the occupational groups. Interestingly, AHR (see Figure 76) is significantly greater during leisure time compared to working time. Contrary to the expectations noted above, we must conclude that emotional load is even higher during leisure time. The significant interaction situation * group obviously is caused by the dispatchers who show rather low AHR at work but relatively high AHR at home. Once more, heart rate variability (see Figure 77) does not differentiate the two situations.

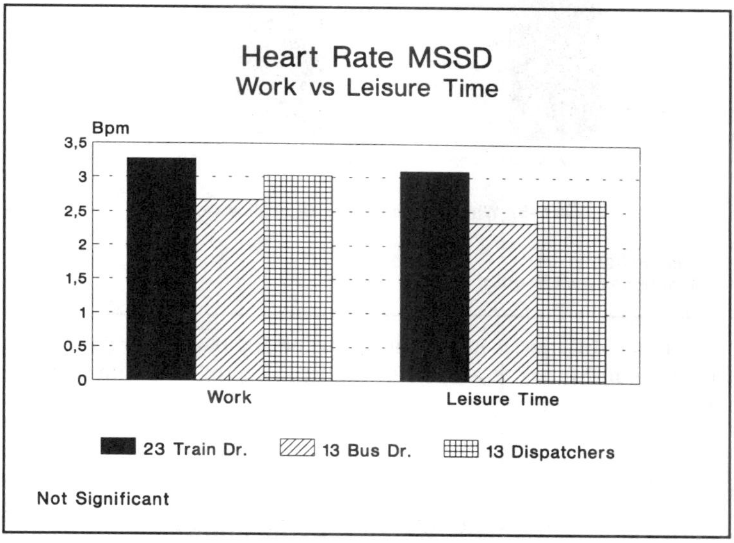

Figure 77. Heart rate variability MSSD in train drivers, bus drivers, and dispatchers during work and leisure time.

Because subjective ratings of excitement and enjoyment were not done during work (only stress ratings on a 3step rating scale), we cannot make the respective comparisons. However, it might be interesting to note the mean values of excitement and enjoyment during leisure time for the three groups. Train drivers rated 1.14 and 1.94, bus drivers 1.16 and 1.90, and dispatchers 1.17 and 1.88 for excitement and enjoyment, respectively.

7.2 Work versus leisure time in white and blue collar workers

In the following, work and leisure time are compared in the blue and white collar workers (sample 17). As already noticed in Chapter 6, heart rate was higher in the blue than in the white collar workers during work (see Figure 78). During leisure time there was no longer a difference. The main effect time and the interaction time * employees are both significant.

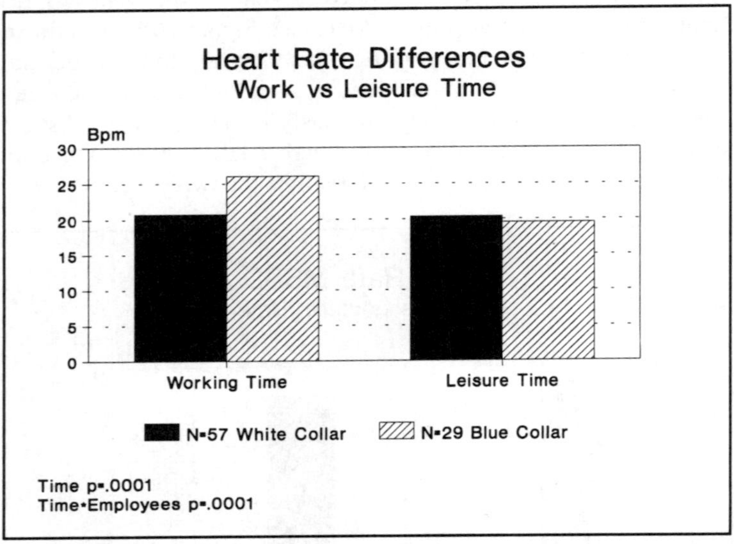

Figure 78. Heart rate (differences to baseline) in white and blue collar workers during work and leisure time. From Myrtek et al., 1999, modified. Reproduced with permission. Copyright 1999 by Elsevier, Oxford.

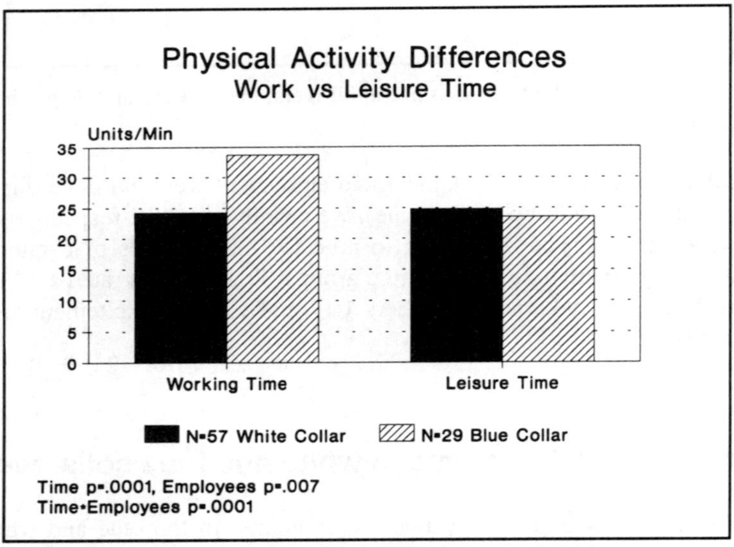

Figure 79. Physical activity (differences to baseline) in white and blue collar workers during work and leisure time. From Myrtek et al., 1999, modified. Reproduced with permission. Copyright 1999 by Elsevier, Oxford.

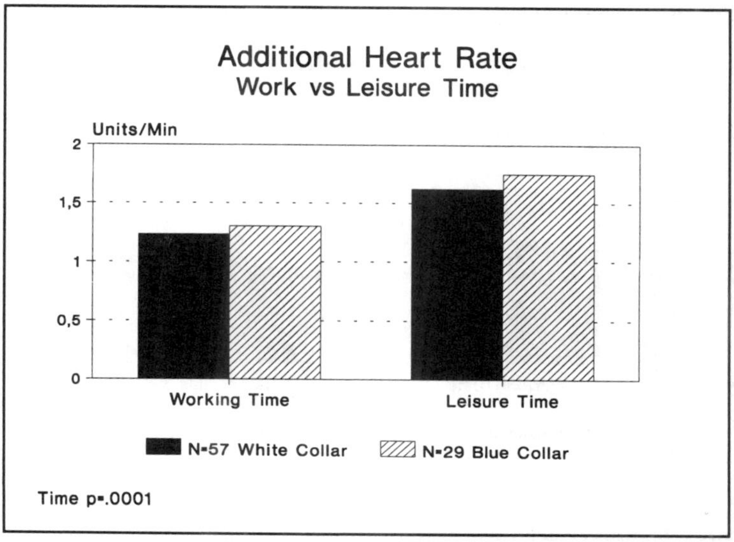

Figure 80. Additional heart rate in white and blue collar workers during work and leisure time. From Myrtek et al., 1999, modified. Reproduced with permission. Copyright 1999 by Elsevier, Oxford.

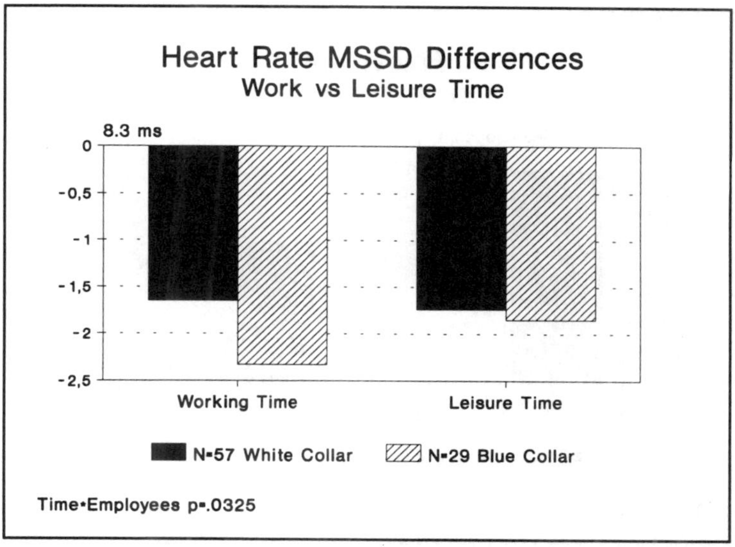

Figure 81. Heart rate variability MSSD (differences to baseline) in white and blue collar workers during work and leisure time. From Myrtek et al., 1999, modified. Reproduced with permission. Copyright 1999 by Elsevier, Oxford.

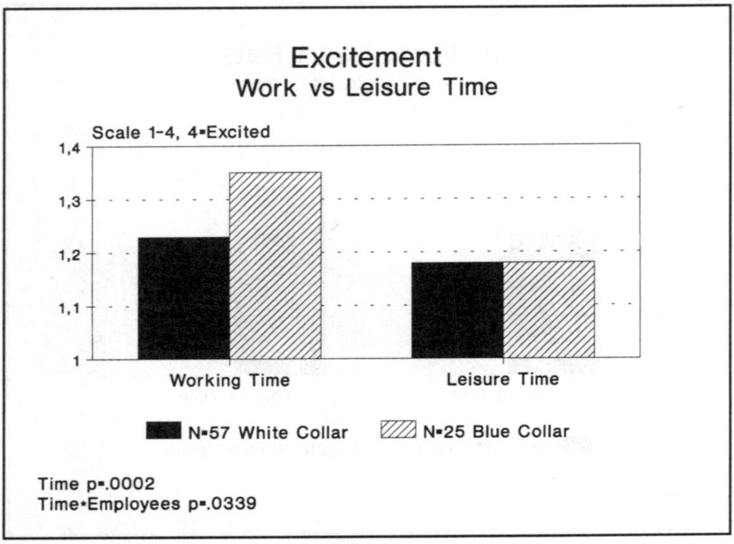

Figure 82. Excitement in white and blue collar workers during work and leisure time. From Myrtek et al., 1999, modified. Reproduced with permission. Copyright 1999 by Elsevier, Oxford.

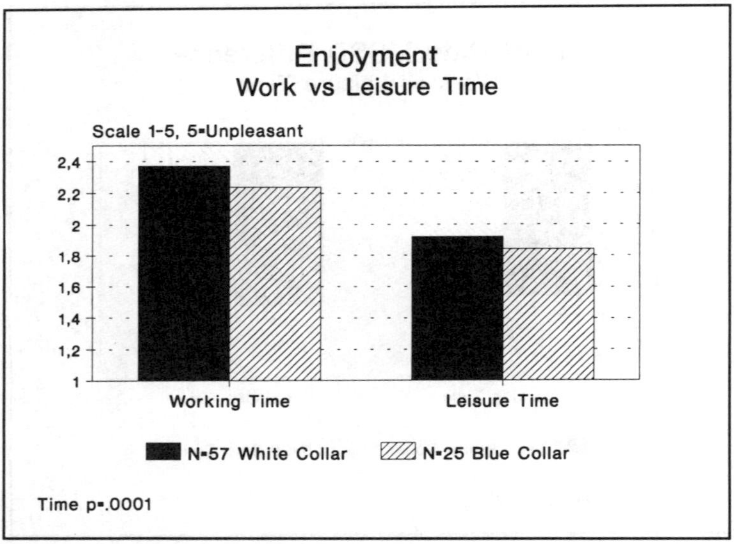

Figure 83. Enjoyment in white and blue collar workers during work and leisure time. From Myrtek et al., 1999, modified. Reproduced with permission. Copyright 1999 by Elsevier, Oxford.

The differences in heart rate are naturally caused by physical activity (see Figure 79) which shows a very similar pattern. The significant differences can be interpreted in the same way as done for heart rate.

AHR (see Figure 80) is significantly higher during leisure time compared to work in both groups. As seen already in the dispatchers as well as the train and bus drivers, emotional work load during leisure time is much higher in blue and white collar workers, too. Heart rate variability (see Figure 81) only shows a significant interaction which is caused by the higher heart rate during work in the blue collar workers. When taking heart rate into account as a covariate, the interaction is no longer significant.

Excitement (see Figure 82) during leisure time, however, is significantly lower than during work in both groups. Blue collar workers were somewhat more excited during work which results in the significant interaction time * employees. For enjoyment (see Figure 83) a significant time effect is observed. Both groups experience less enjoyment during work as compared to leisure time.

When we look at the figures for excitement and enjoyment during leisure time in train and bus drivers, dispatchers, as well as blue and white collar workers we notice a great similarity between all occupational groups.

7.3 Effects of television viewing in schoolboys

In the study with schoolboys (Myrtek & Scharff, 2000; sample 6 and 7), we were especially interested in possible effects of television viewing because a good deal of the leisure time is devoted to TV. With the feedbacks of the FMS, it was possible to estimate the time of TV viewing very exactly. Each sample was split at the median in light and heavy TV viewers. Of the 50 11-year-old boys with light consumption, six boys did not watch TV at all on the day of recording, and of the 50 15-year-old boys with light consumption seven boys did not watch TV. Therefore, the columns in the Figures represent 44, 50, 43, and 50 boys, respectively. The younger boys watched on average 1.85 hours on normal schooldays and the older boys 2.29 hours. Younger boys with light TV consumption watched 0.78 hours the older boys with light consumption 1.10 hours. The respective figures for boys with heavy TV consumption are 2.92 and 3.28 hours.

In the following Figures, we compare schooltime with TV-time at home. Heart rate (see Figure 84) naturally is lower during TV viewing because physical activity (see Figure 85) is low in this situation. The significant interaction stay * TV denotes that light TV consumers have a higher heart rate during viewing TV, although differences at school are not so distinct. The threefold interaction stay * age * TV is obviously caused by the older boys. At school their heart rate was highest and during TV viewing heart rate was low. Clearly, this is not caused by physical activity. Physical activity is generally higher in the younger boys than in the older. The interaction stay * age denotes that the younger boys compared to the older show higher physical activity at school but during TV watching there is no clear difference between the age groups.

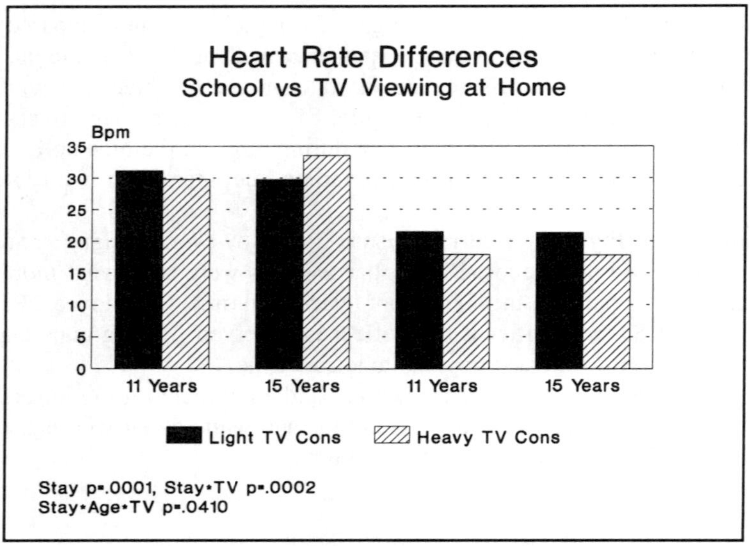

Figure 84. Heart rate (differences to baseline) at school and during TV viewing at home in schoolboys From Myrtek & Scharff, 2000, modified. Reproduced with permission. Copyright 2000 by Huber, Bern.

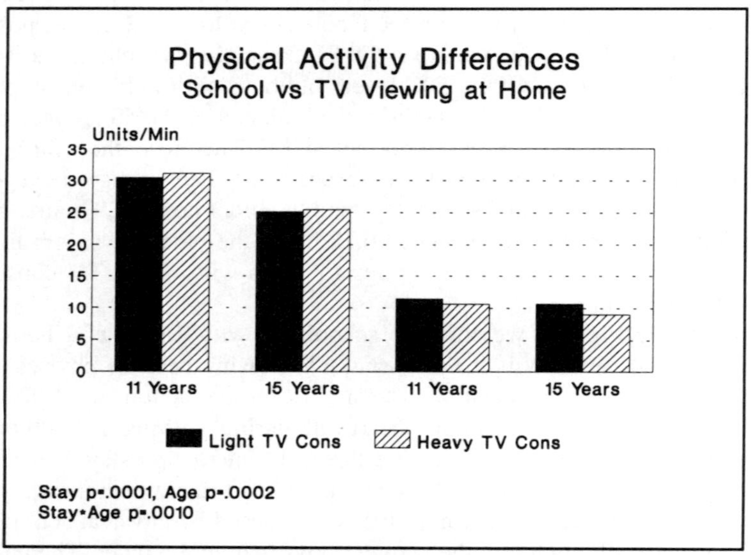

Figure 85. Physical activity (differences to baseline) at school and during TV viewing at home in schoolboys. From Myrtek & Scharff, 2000, modified. Reproduced with permission. Copyright 2000 by Huber, Bern.

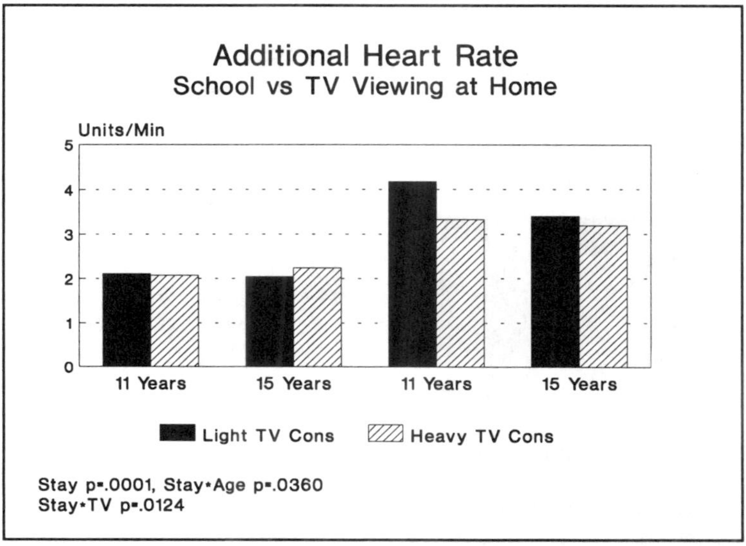

Figure 86. Additional heart rate at school and during TV viewing at home in schoolboys. From Myrtek & Scharff, 2000, modified. Reproduced with permission. Copyright 2000 by Huber, Bern.

Especially relevant is the high difference in AHR (see Figure 86). At school, AHR is rather low in all groups but during TV viewing AHR is high. The interaction stay * age denotes that AHR is not very different between the age groups at school but during TV viewing AHR is higher in the younger than in the older group. Finally, AHR is dependent on the amount of TV consumption as indicated by the interaction stay * TV. As already stated, the group differences at school are not distinct but during TV viewing boys with light consumption show higher AHR than boys with heavy consumption. This means that the emotional impact of TV consumption becomes lower with higher consumption.

Heart rate variability was lower at school compared to watching TV (see Figure 87). The interaction stay * TV means that boys with heavy consumption show lower variability at school. However, after adjusting for heart rate these differences are no longer significant.

As might be expected, excitement was rated as lower during TV viewing than during time at school (see Figure 88). The threefold interaction stay * age * TV denotes that older boys with heavy TV consumption rated more excitement at school compared to the younger boys with heavy consumption whereas the other groups showed no differences. Enjoyment also revealed a significant difference (see Figure 89). TV viewing was rated to be more pleasant than staying at school. Older boys enjoyed school even less than younger boys as indicated by the interaction stay * age. Again, a threefold interaction was observed which can be interpreted in the same way as for excitement.

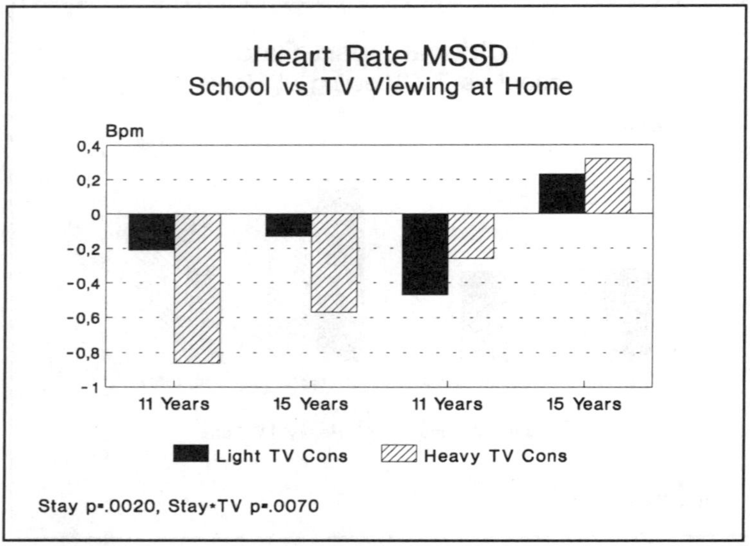

Figure 87. Heart rate variability MSSD (differences to baseline) at school and during TV viewing at home in schoolboys From Myrtek & Scharff, 2000, modified. Reproduced with permission. Copyright 2000 by Huber, Bern.

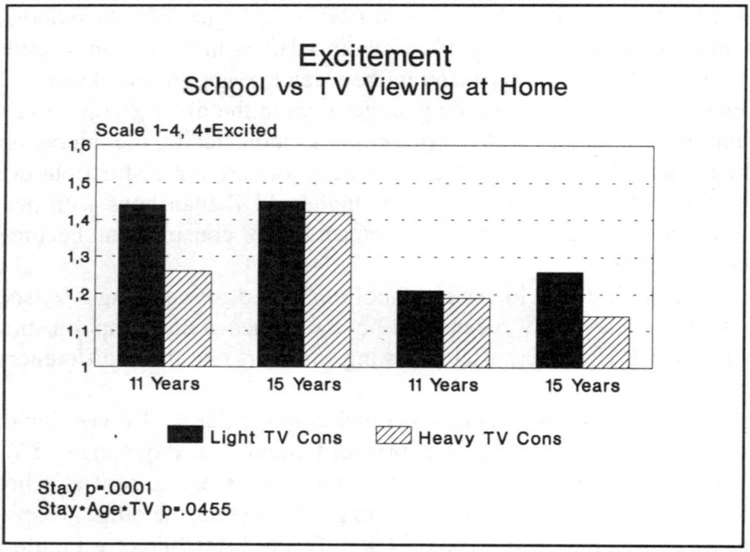

Figure 88. Excitement at school and during TV viewing at home in schoolboys. From Myrtek & Scharff, 2000, modified. Reproduced with permission. Copyright 2000 by Huber, Bern.

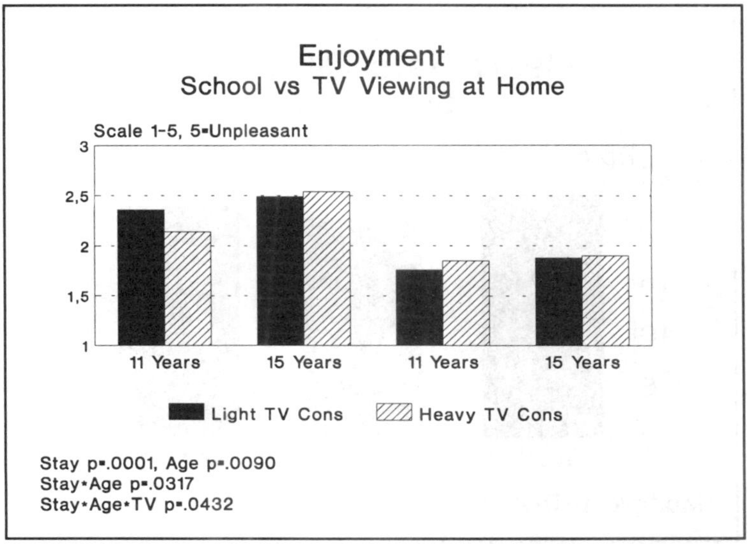

Figure 89. Enjoyment at school and during TV viewing at home in schoolboys. From Myrtek & Scharff, 2000, modified. Reproduced with permission. Copyright 2000 by Huber, Bern.

7.4 Driving a car

One of the main activities in daily life is driving a car. This is mostly done during leisure time or to get to the workplace. There are high levels of traffic and congestion on the streets. In the small country of Germany with 82 million inhabitants there are about 45 million private cars. Accidents with injuries and even deaths are frequent. Therefore, it is conceivable that driving a car ought to be highly stressful. We would expect a higher emotional work load in these situations compared to other situations of daily life.

7.4.1 White and blue collar workers

Of the 106 white and blue collar workers (sample 17), 65 drove a car during monitoring with the FMS. We will compare the following situations: Work, leisure time, and driving a car. Driving a car was on the average 14 minutes and short compared to the other situations.

Heart rate during leisure time (see Figure 90) is lower than during working time ($p = .008$); the other comparisons with the t test are not significant. Physical activity (see Figure 91) was high during driving compared to work and leisure time (both p values $< .001$) and lowest during leisure time ($p = .011$ compared to work).

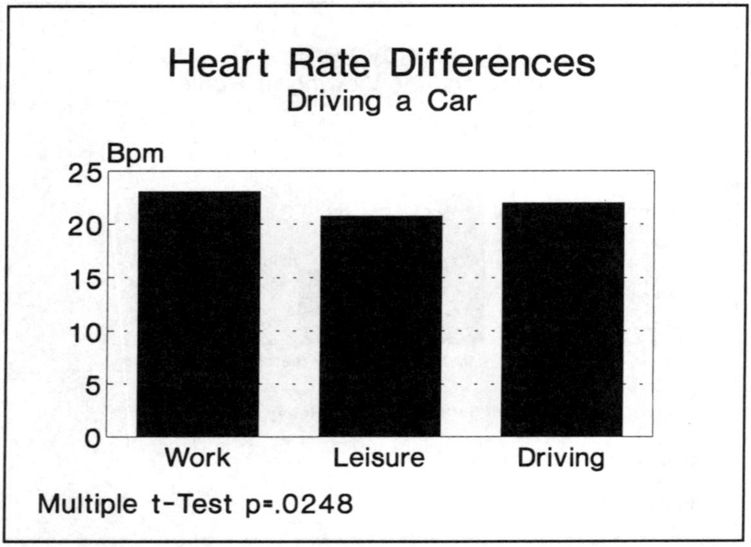

Figure 90. Heart rate (differences to baseline) at work, during leisure time, and during car driving in blue and white collar workers.

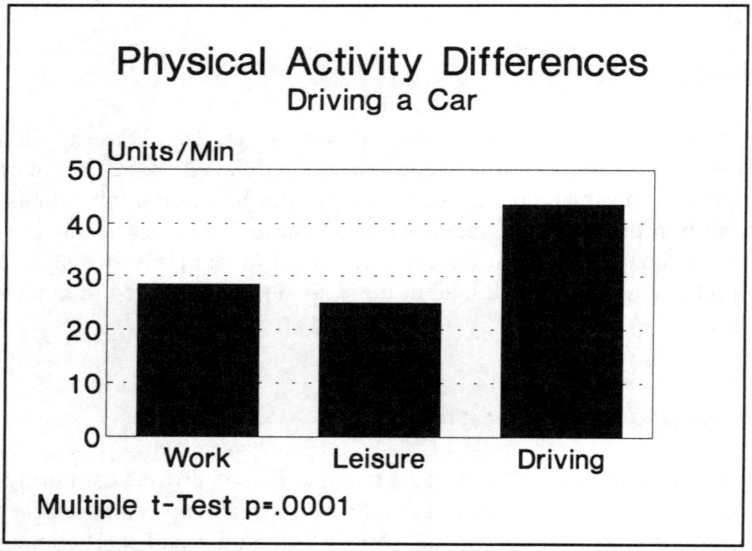

Figure 91. Physical activity (differences to baseline) at work, during leisure time, and during car driving in blue and white collar workers.

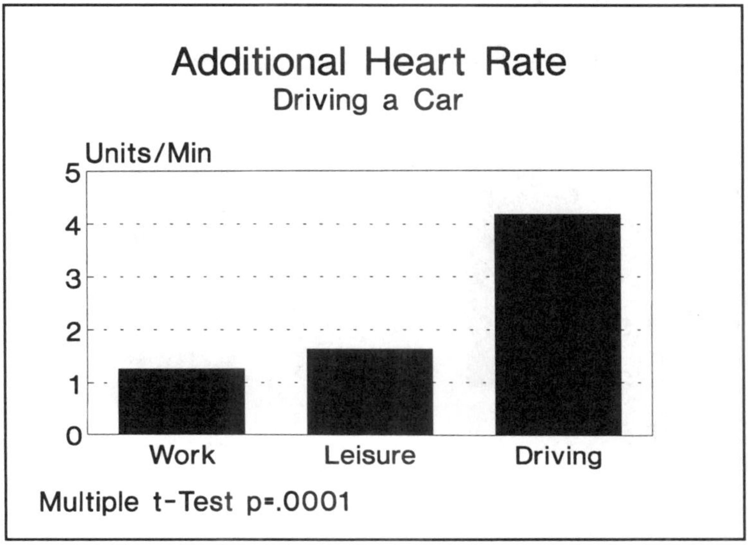

Figure 92. Additional heart rate at work, during leisure time, and during car driving in blue and white collar workers.

There are several explanations for the high physical activity during driving in this group compared to the students in Chapter 7.4.2. First, the segment of driving varied between 3 and 68 minutes with an average of 14 minutes whereas in the students this segment was nearly constant at 32 minutes. Therefore, carry over effects from other physical activities might have heightened the activity in the blue and white collar workers such as getting in and getting out of the car which is not as crucial in the long driving segment of the students. Second, drivers in the workers group had to handle the feedbacks by themselves which is not quite so simple during driving, whereas in the case of the students the front-seat passenger handled the FMS for the driver. Finally, it is known from the students examination that driving in town demands more physical activity than driving on a main road or express-way. The most important result is the high AHR (see Figure 92) during driving indicating high emotional or mental work load. Compared to both, work and leisure time, AHR was significantly greater during driving (both p values < .001). There was also a significant difference between work and leisure time ($p < .001$) as already reported in Chapter 7.2. Heart rate variability (see Figure 93) was not significantly different.
Excitement (see Figure 94) was highest during driving and the difference between driving and leisure time was significant ($p = .004$). No significant difference between driving and work was observed. Excitement was also greater during work than during leisure time ($p = .017$). Nearly the same pattern was seen for enjoyment (see Figure 95). Leisure time was rated to be more pleasant than work or driving (both p values < .001).

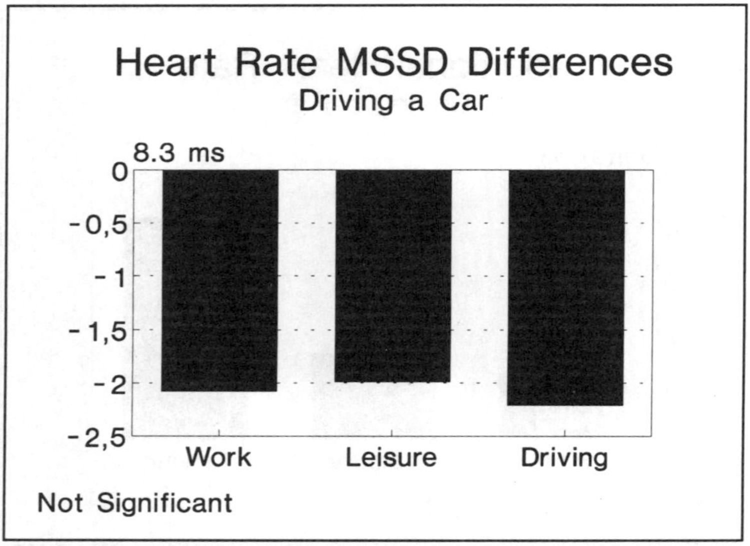

Figure 93. Heart rate variability MSSD (differences to baseline) at work, during leisure time, and during car driving in blue and white collar workers.

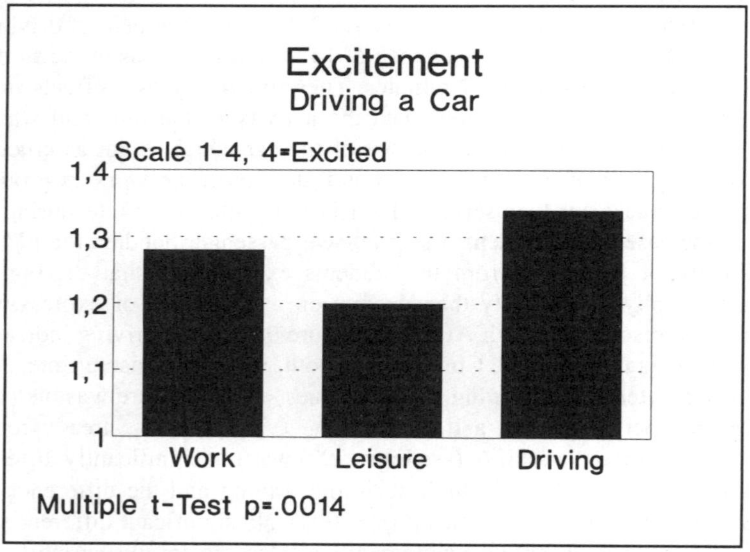

Figure 94. Excitement at work, during leisure time, and during car driving in blue and white collar workers.

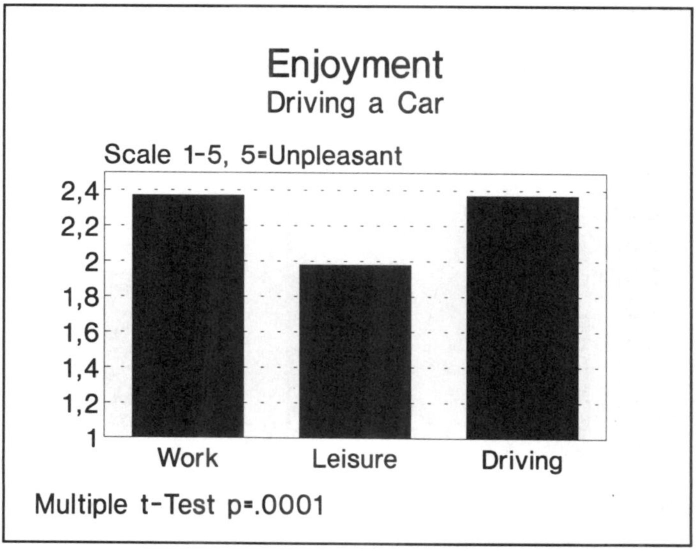

Figure 95. Enjoyment at work, during leisure time, and during car driving in blue and white collar workers.

7.4.2 Male university students

Forty male university students (mean age 24.7 years; sample 14) were monitored with the FMS during their car drive to a large amusement park about 36 km away from their university town (Piech, 2002). Together with the experimenter, two subjects at the time traveled to the park. One subject drove the car on the way there, the other subject drove the car back. In this way we can compare active with passive driving. Moreover, the values measured during the whole day (values for driving included) are given for comparison.

Heart rate response (see Figure 96) was significantly greater during active driving than during passive driving ($p < .001$) or during the whole day ($p = .003$). This heart rate response was not caused by physical activity (see Figure 97). On the contrary, physical activity was significantly lower both during active and passive driving (both p values $< .001$). The front-seat passengers also showed higher physical activity than the active drivers ($p = .009$).

According to the pattern with high heart rate and low physical activity, AHR was greatest for the active drivers compared to the passengers ($p < .001$) and compared to the whole day ($p = .001$). AHR for the passengers was also significantly lower ($p < .001$) than during the whole day (see Figure 98). Heart rate variability (see Figure 99) also showed significant differences but after adjusting for heart rate the multiple t test was no longer significant.

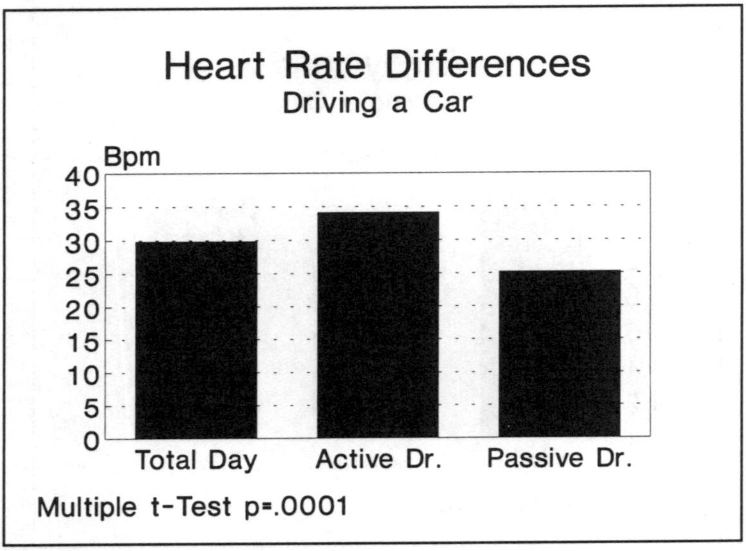

Figure 96. Heart rate (differences to baseline) during the total daytime, active driving, and passive driving in students.

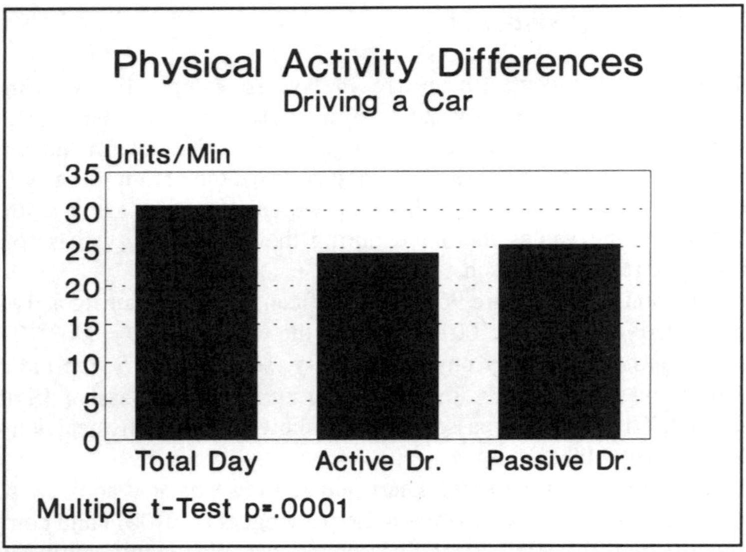

Figure 97. Physical activity (differences to baseline) during the total daytime, active driving, and passive driving in students.

Both excitement (see Figure 100) and enjoyment (see Figure 101) revealed no significant differences. This clearly contradicts the notion that excitement or enjoyment ratings are perceptions of the actual physiological state.

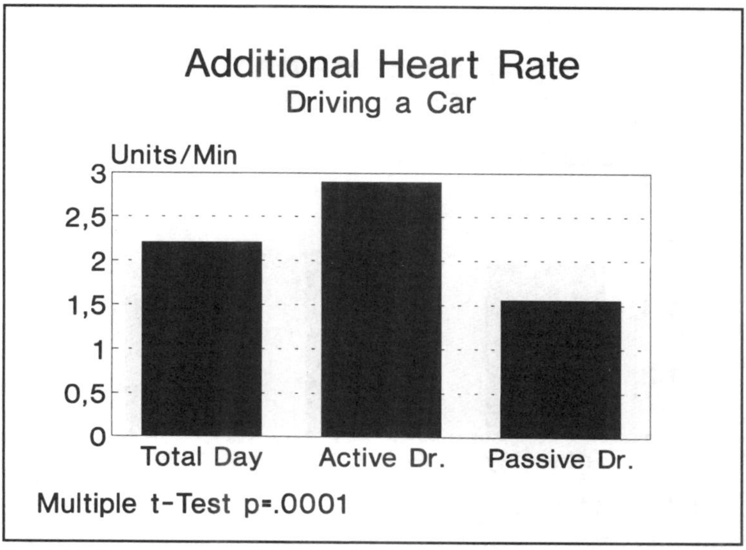

Figure 98. Additional heart rate during the total daytime, active driving, and passive driving in students.

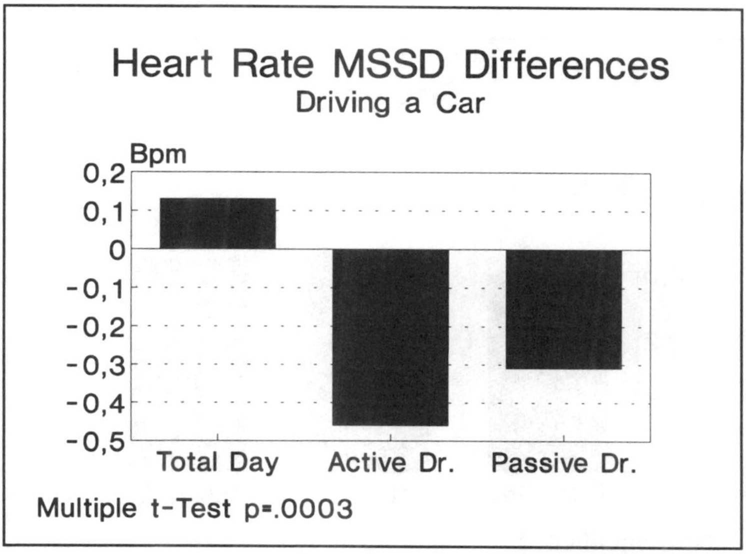

Figure 99. Heart rate variability MSSD (differences to baseline) during the total daytime, active driving, and passive driving in students.

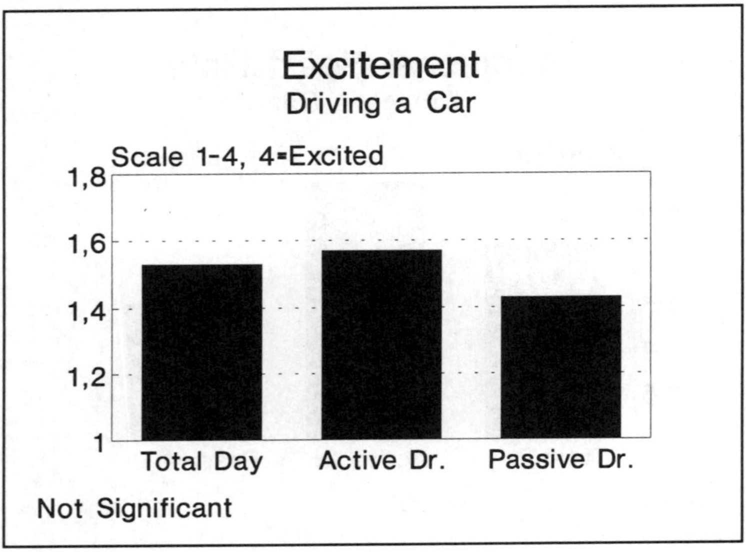

Figure 100. Excitement during the total daytime, active driving, and passive driving in students.

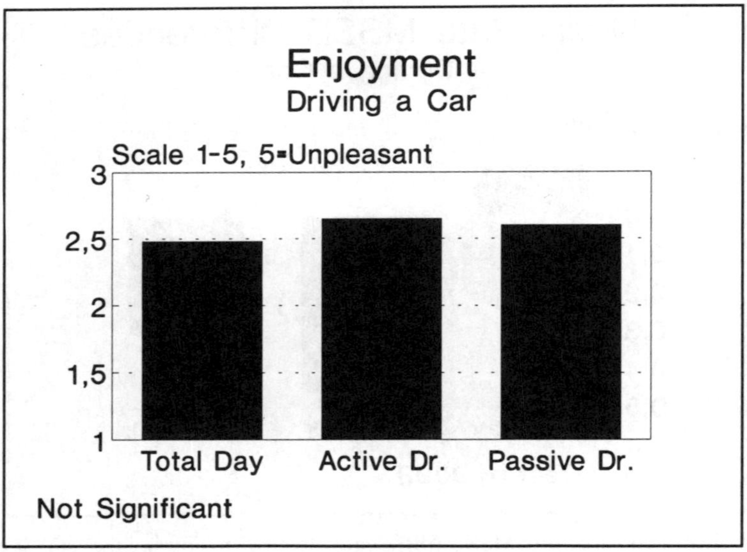

Figure 101. Enjoyment during the total daytime, active driving, and passive driving in students.

7.5 Stress at the amusement park

As stated above, students drove to an amusement park. Here, subjects visited the following attractions in permutated order: Rafting, driving up the "Eurotower," riding the roller coaster "Mir," and riding a big swingboat. Rafting is very harmless and relaxing. One sits on a wooden raft pulled slowly through a small lake which is lined along the shore with different adventure scenes. Driving up the 70 m tower, too, was harmless, except for those predisposed to aerophobia. The roller coaster was rather exciting, with an acceleration of 3.3 g downwards. Most exciting, however, was the swingboat. In the following, these attractions and the values of the whole day are compared with one another.

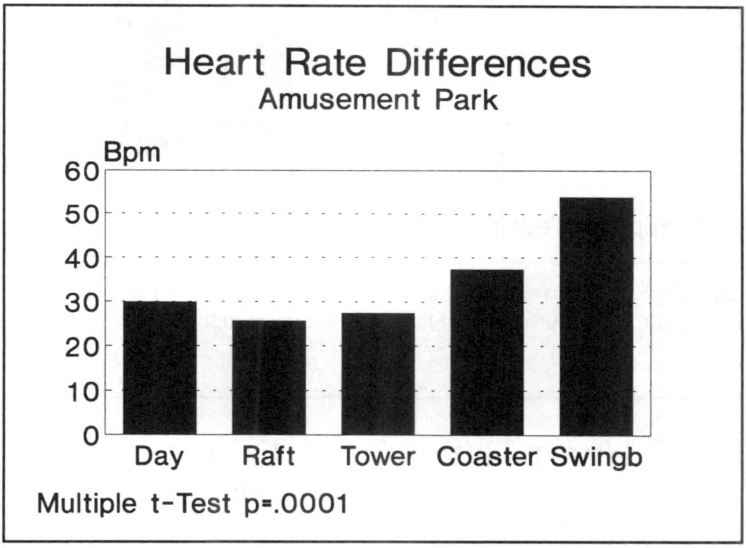

Figure 102. Heart rate (differences to baseline) in students during total daytime and several attractions of an amusement park: Raft, Eurotower, roller coaster, and swingboat.

Heart rate responses on the swingboat were extremely high with an average of more than 54 bpm over baseline values (see Figure 102). All comparisons with the other attractions and the whole day are highly significant ($p < .001$). The roller coaster, too, caused high heart rate responses with significant differences compared to the other situations ($p < .001$). Driving up the Eurotower produced a moderate heart rate response. The comparison with the whole day is not significant but response on the tower was greater than that during rafting ($p = .021$). The lowest heart rate was observed during rafting. Compared to the whole day, response during rafting is significantly lower ($p < .001$).

Physical activity is not presented here because the differences in the activities do not reflect real physical activity. The physical activities on the swingboat, the roller coaster, and the tower were also not suitable for the computation of AHR. Therefore, we decided to substitute these activities by the activity subjects' showed during passive driving as a front-seat passenger.

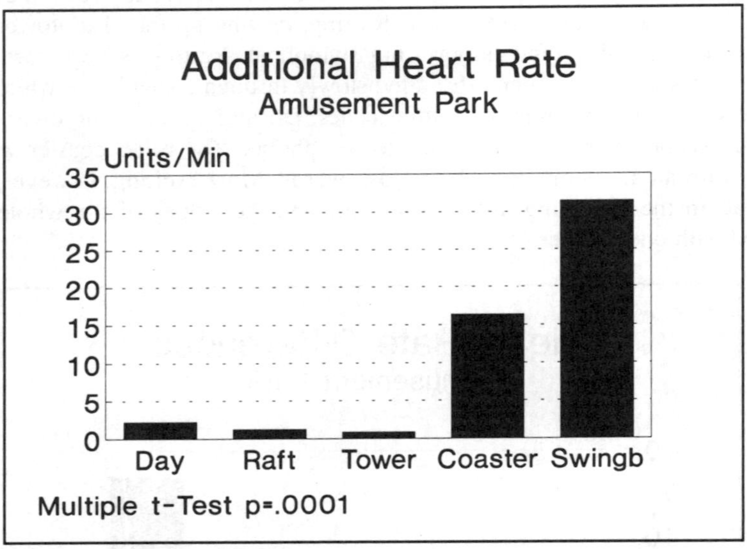

Figure 103. Additional heart rate in students during total daytime and several attractions of an amusement park: Raft, Eurotower, roller coaster, and swingboat.

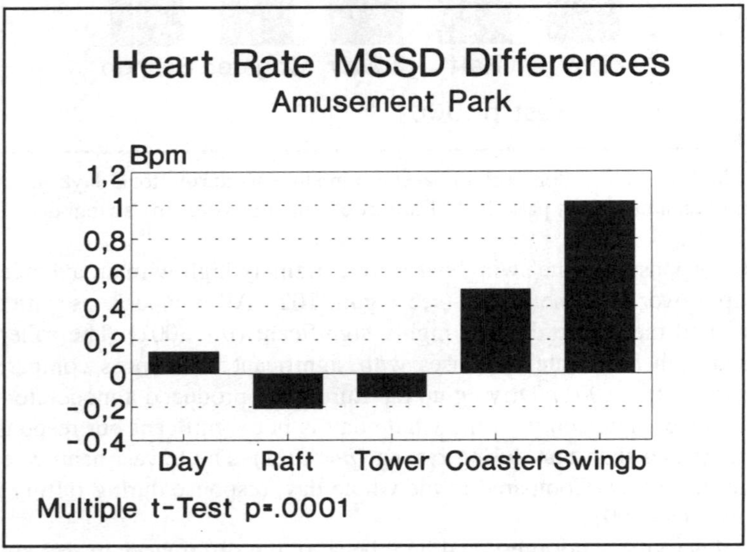

Figure 104. Heart rate variability MSSD (differences to baseline) in students during total daytime and several attractions of an amusement park: Raft, Eurotower, roller coaster, and swingboat.

The up and downs of the swingboat produced high variations of heart rate and, therefore, produced extremely high values for AHR (see Figure 103) with significant differences compared to the other situations ($p < .001$). AHR on the roller coaster is high also and, with the exception of the swingboat, all AHR values are greater than in the other situations ($p < .001$). As might be expected, AHR during rafting and driving up the tower is low with no significant difference. AHR on the tower and during rafting is significantly lower than AHR of the whole day ($p = .002$ and $p < .001$). Heart rate variability (see Figure 104) also showed significant differences with higher values for the swingboat and the roller coaster. However, these responses are contrary to what we expected. According to these figures, mental work load would be even lower during these situations. Therefore, we will not further interpret these data.

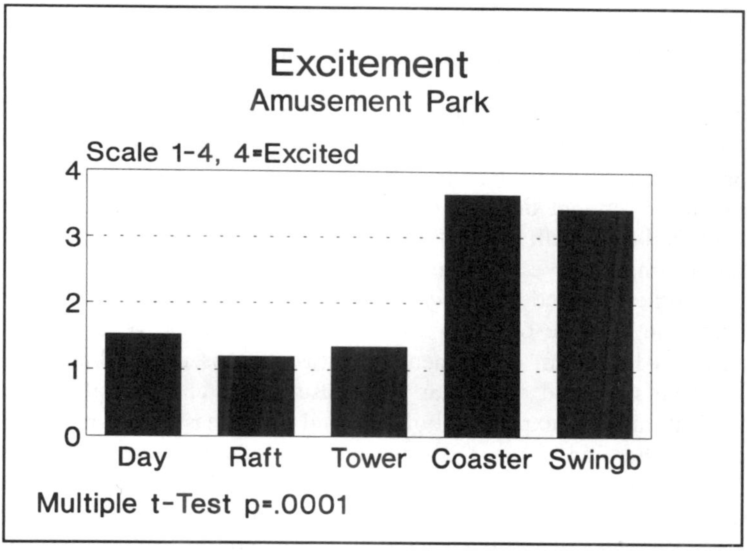

Figure 105. Excitement in students during total daytime and several attractions of an amusement park: Raft, Eurotower, roller coaster, and swingboat.

During the attractions tower, roller coaster, and swingboat we switched off the feedback signals. Answering questions presented on a display is of course very difficult when riding on a roller coaster. However, subjects were asked about their excitement after each attraction. Excitement (see Figure 105) was rated to be very high on both the roller coaster and the swingboat with no significant difference between these situations. Compared to the other situations, all differences for excitement are significant ($p < .001$). Excitement was, however, low during rafting and on the tower with no significant difference. Compared to the whole day, both rafting and driving up the tower showed lower excitement ($p < .001$ and $p = .030$).

7.6 Discussion

As this Chapter has shown, leisure time can be more stressful than work and some activities such as driving a car are especially stressful. In all groups, train drivers, bus drivers, and dispatchers, AHR was higher at home than at work indicating higher emotional work load during leisure time. We have indications that certain situations such as sitting at the table together with the family during supper produce far more AHR than for instance reading the newspaper. We can imagine what is going on in such situations. The children tell of their marks at school which perhaps are not the best, the wife is complaining of not having enough housekeeping money, etc. The observation of a higher AHR during leisure time than during work is also substantiated by our sample of blue and white collar workers. Nevertheless, the workers rate excitement to be lower during leisure time than during work and that they enjoy leisure time far more than work. It is obvious that these ratings are not based on a perception of the bodily state but are cognitive schemas as already stated in Chapters 4 and 5.

Our studies with schoolboys have shown that especially TV viewing elicits emotional load. Again this load is not perceived by the boys, because viewing TV is rated to be more pleasant and less exciting than staying at school. The emotional load is dependent on the amount of former TV viewing. Older boys are not so impressed than younger and boys with heavy TV consumption do not respond as much as boys with light consumption. We might interpret this attenuation of emotional reactivity as emotional bluntness caused by heavy TV consumption. However, this interpretation is an assumption because our data are correlational. To prove causal relationship would require a long-term experiment with two groups of children, whereby one group would be subjected to regular TV consumption and the other group to TV abstinence. Naturally, an experiment of this kind is not feasible for many reasons. On the other hand there are several reasons in favor of our interpretation. Boys with heavy TV consumption did not show differences in AHR or heart rate itself during total leisure time or during school time, thus limiting the finding of reduced AHR and reduced heart rate itself to the time of TV consumption.

Zillmann and Bryant (1982) conducted an experiment with four student groups with 20 subjects each of which were subjected to different doses of pornographic movies over six weeks: Six pornographic movies, three pornographic and three neutral movies, six neutral movies, and no movie at all. After nine weeks from the beginning of the experiment, subjects were asked to disclose their attitudes toward unusual sexual habits, permissiveness to show erotic movies on the TV, etc. The attitudes of the students were dependent on the number of pornographic movies they had seen. Students of the first two groups believed that unusual sexual habits are more prevalent in the population and were more permissive towards erotic movies on TV than the other groups. In a second study by Zillmann and Bryant (1988) with 80 students and 80 other adults, the effect of a sexual bluntness was substantiated. After the experiment, subjects in the pornographic as compared to the non-pornographic groups were less satisfied with their partners, the appearance of their partners, etc.

Cline, Croft, and Courrier (1973) exposed 80 five to 12-year-old boys with light or heavy TV consumption to a moderately violent movie. Before and during the exposure, blood volume pulse amplitudes were measured. Children with heavy TV consumption were significantly less aroused than children with light consumption. In a second experiment with 40 other boys, skin conductance and blood volume pulse amplitude were measured. The findings of the first study were replicated. In an experiment with 44 boys and girls (age 8 to 10 years) it was also shown that children who had seen more TV violence showed lower reactivity in skin resistance when viewing a videotaped scene of real aggression (Hanratty-Thomas, Horton, Lippincott, & Drabman, 1977).

In a study with six-year-old preschool children, 18 boys and 18 girls were recorded with the FMS in their home environment while viewing different television films (Wilhelm, Myrtek, & Brügner, 1997). Two cartoons designed for children of this age and a sequence of commercials were presented in a balanced order. One cartoon consisted of many action scenes ("Ghostbusters") the other reported the story of "Unlucky Jack". Heart rate and additional heart rate were significantly higher for Ghostbusters than for Unlucky Jack, the commercials appearing between both cartoons. Generally, girls displayed higher heart rate than boys, but during Ghostbusters heart rate was higher in boys. For the commercials, a significant interaction sex * type of commercial was found. Girls' heart rate was higher for commercials designed for girls (e.g., Barbie) than for sex neutral commercials (e.g., Smarties). Children with light TV consumption (rated by their parents) showed significantly more AHR than children with heavy TV consumption.

The point of emotional bluntness through heavy TV consumption is so important because it might be that bluntness is transferred to real life situations. Johnson, Cohen, Smailes, Kasen, and Brook (2002) assessed the amount of TV viewing and aggressive behavior over a 17-year interval in a sample of 707 persons. The amount of time spent watching TV during adolescence and early adulthood, was associated with subsequent aggressive acts against other persons. Aggressive acts increased with increasing time of TV viewing and was lowest when consumption was below one hour per day. The authors controlled for several factors which might have been influenced the result: Childhood neglect, family income, previous aggressive behavior, etc. The result, however, remained significant. It is possible that the link between the amount of TV consumption and later aggressive acts is really the reduction of emotional reactivity through heavy TV consumption as observed in our studies.

Although driving a car is a common activity for most people, only little research is done on this issue. Most of the research is made with simulated car driving (e.g., Musante et al., 2000; Roge, Pebayle, & Muzet, 2001) or with special groups such as car racing drivers (Schwaberger, 1987). However, as shown by Wilson (2001) in studies with aircraft pilots, simulation cannot mimic real flight situations. Taggart, Gibbons, and Somerville (1969) examined 32 experienced car drivers (mean age 29 years, range 21 to 55) while driving their own cars in London traffic for about 20 minutes. Average heart rate during driving was 98 bpm with a wide variation between 70 and 145 bpm. This variation in heart rate caused by the changing traffic situations are the reason for the high AHR observed in our driver samples. In the blue and white collar workers, AHR was much greater during driving than during the working hours. However, driving was rated to be equally exciting and pleasant than working. Similar results were observed for students driving to the amusement park. In this study, a differentiation was made between active and passive driving. As shown by AHR, active driving was far more stressful than passive driving.

Finally, we examined the stress in an amusement park. Millions of people visit such parks every year but nearly nothing is known about the physiological effects of riding a roller coaster or a swingboat. The search in the literature did not produce any information; obviously no research on this subject has been done. We only found a short notice by Pringle, Macfarlane, and Cobbe (1989). These authors examined a roller coaster ride in seven women and six men with a mean age of 28 years with ambulatory electrocardiography. The acceleration force of the coaster was 3 g and in the same range as the coaster in our amusement park. Mean heart rate increased from 70 bpm before the ride to 154 bpm during it. The authors were impressed by the observation that all subjects reached their maximum heart rate in less than eight seconds. Compared to our students who showed an average increase of 37 bpm above baseline, the observed 84 bpm on the coaster in Glasgow are much greater. Presumably, this also depends on the sample because in the Glasgow study more than the half were women. Excitement was rated by our students to be rather high in both roller coaster and swingboat but did not differentiate these attractions. From a physiological point of view, the swingboat clearly revealed the greatest total and emotional work load.

7.7 Summary

This Chapter was devoted to stressful situations encountered during leisure time. The working time of the train drivers, bus drivers, and dispatchers was compared to their leisure time. In all groups, AHR was significantly greater during leisure time, indicating higher emotional work load at home. This result was replicated by the findings made in the blue and white collar workers. Despite these facts, leisure time was rated to be more enjoyable and less exciting than staying at work.

In our studies with schoolboys, we were interested in possible effects of TV viewing in the home environment as compared to school time. TV viewing was emotionally far more stressful than school time as indicated by AHR. However, staying at school was rated as more exciting and less pleasant than viewing TV. A most interesting result was that AHR was dependent on the amount of watching TV. Boys with heavy TV consumption showed lower AHR compared to boys with light consumption. The same was true for older as compared to younger boys. This finding was interpreted as emotional bluntness, presumably caused by the amount of TV consumption. Although this assumption cannot ultimately be proven by our study, we have several good reasons for this interpretation.

In everyday life, driving a car is as normal as sleeping or eating. Most drivers are convinced that driving a car is not very stressful, except during stop and go. However, AHR was much greater during driving than during the working hours in blue and white collar workers, indicating high emotional work load. This result was substantiated by our students during active driving to an amusement park. Both groups were not able to perceive the high emotional load correctly because excitement or enjoyment were not rated differently compared to the working hours in blue and white collar workers or the total daytime in students.

Our last sample for stress during leisure time stems from an amusement park. Our students were submitted to rides on a roller coaster and a big swingboat. Heart rate and AHR were extremely high during both attractions, especially on the swingboat, indicating high total and emotional work load. Subjective ratings of the excitement during these attractions compared to other more harmless attractions were somewhat in line with the physiological indicators but did not differentiate the roller coaster from the swingboat.

Chapter 8

Physiological monitoring during the night

Monitoring during sleep was used in order to establish a proper baseline. However, monitoring at night might offer further interesting information, e.g., comparing subjects with to subjects without sleep disturbances. In our studies, we routinely assessed certain personality dimensions, physical complaints, and life habits as well as anamnestic data, with questionnaires. One question in the anamnestic data sheet pertains to sleep disturbances on a five point scale with the frequencies "never," "about once a month," "about once a week," "about three times a week," and "nearly everyday." In patients (samples 02 and 04) we combined the ratings "never" and "about once a month" to represent normal sleep. The combination of the other ratings represented disturbed sleep. In the female students (samples 08 and 12), the category "never sleep disturbances" was contrasted with the other categories.

8.1 Hypotheses

As shown by Pivik and Busby (1996) in 21 children, sleep onset is accompanied by a decrease in heart rate. In a second study with 14 preadolescents it was also found that heart rate decreased across the initial four sleep cycles (Pivik, Busby, Gill, Hunter, & Nevins, 1996). Heart rate during rapid eye movement sleep (REM) was significantly higher than during non-rapid eye movement sleep (NREM). In eight healthy adults, a continuous decrease of heart rate during the night was observed in both REM as well as NREM (Cajochen, Pischke, Aeschbach, & Borbely, 1994). This study also confirmed the observation that heart rate was greater during REM as opposed to NREM in every sleep cycle. During the transition from NREM to REM heart rate increase was rapid whereas the decline from REM to NREM was slow.

An increase in heart rate and heart rate variability during REM was also observed by Zemaityte, Varoneckas, and Sokolov (1984) in 20 healthy men. During NREM stages 3 and 4, heart rate was about 52 bpm and increased to 55 bpm during REM. In another study by Van de Borne et al. (1995) with 13 healthy men, an increase from 50 bpm (NREM-3 and 4) to 55 bpm was found.

According to these studies, we would expect a decline in heart rate during the night. Clearly, sudden increases of heart rate during REM will produce AHR during these stages. Because it is known from many studies that the duration of the REM stages increases during the night, we would also expect an increase in AHR. Moreover, a decrease in physical activity would be expected because sleep onset is most likely not as calm as later sleep periods.

Bonnet and Arand (1998) compared 12 insomniacs with 12 healthy controls, matched for age, sex, and body weight. In the former group, heart rate was increased by about 7 bpm. Spectral analysis revealed increased low frequency power and decreased high frequency power in insomniacs compared to controls. This means that insomniacs show higher sympathetic and lower parasympathetic nervous system activity. In addition, subjective total sleeping time was reduced in insomniacs compared to controls. In a study by Martinez-Lavin, Hermosillo, Rosas, and Soto (1998), 30 patients with rheumatic diseases and sleep disturbances were compared to 30 healthy controls matched for age and sex. There were no heart rate differences between the groups but spectral analysis revealed a predominance of the low-frequency band (LF/HF ratio) indicating an exaggerated sympathetic modulation of the sinus node in the patients. A higher sympathetic activity during sleep was also observed in 29 patients with panic disorder compared to 23 healthy controls (Yeragani et al., 1998). This result was also confirmed by Sloan et al. (1999) in 24 patients with panic disorder and 12 healthy controls. According to these results in the literature, we would expect higher heart rate and shorter sleeping time in our sleep disturbed groups. Moreover, the higher sympathetic activation in subjects with sleep disturbances might cause more AHR and more depression of the ST-segment amplitude. Finally, there might be a higher physical activity during the night in subjects with sleep disturbances.

It is known from our former studies (Myrtek, 1998a) that subjects with sleep disturbances also complain more frequently about other physical symptoms and often reveal greater emotional lability in personality questionnaires. Therefore, we would expect higher emotional lability and more bodily complaints in subjects with sleep disturbances.

8.2 Results

Indeed, subjects with sleep disturbances were tested and found to be emotionally more labile than good sleepers in all groups (p = .001 to p =.046). In the patient groups, bad sleepers also significantly rated bodily complaints more frequently (both p values = .001). During feedback they also complained of having more angina pectoris (p = .008 and p = .033). In patients with disturbed sleep, the consumption of sleeping tablets and tranquilizers was also significantly greater than in the normal patient groups (both p values < .050). However, sleeping time as assessed by the time during which the feedback algorithm was turned off, was not significantly different in good and poor sleepers of the patient groups and in one student group. In the first student group, subjects with sleep disturbances even slept about 50 minutes longer. In the following Figures, we present hourly values for the first seven hours of the night. Sleep onset was defined by turning off the feedback algorithm on going to bed.

Heart rate continuously dropped during the night in all groups and was lowest in the seventh hour. For the cardiac patients, there was a tendency for heart rate in patients with sleep disturbances to be somewhat higher (p = .089; see Figures 106 to 109).

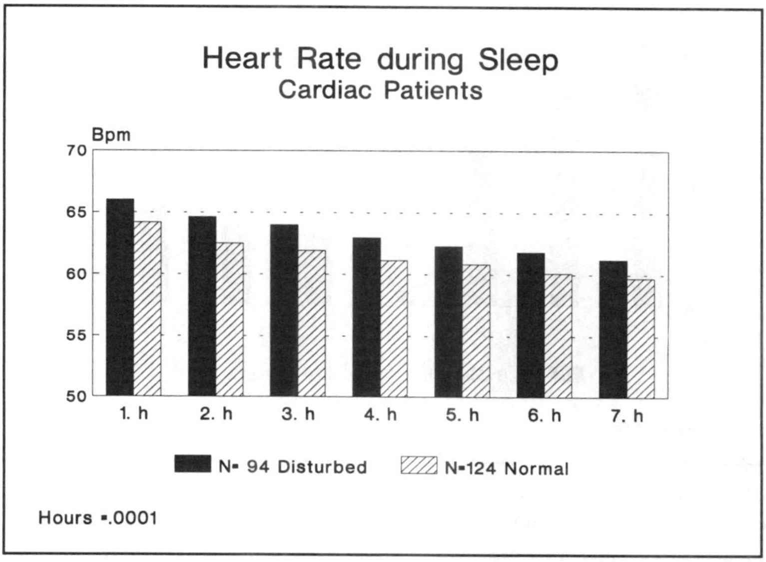

Figure 106. Heart rate during sleep in cardiac patients. From Myrtek, 2002, modified. Reproduced with permission. Copyright 2002 by Hogrefe, Göttingen.

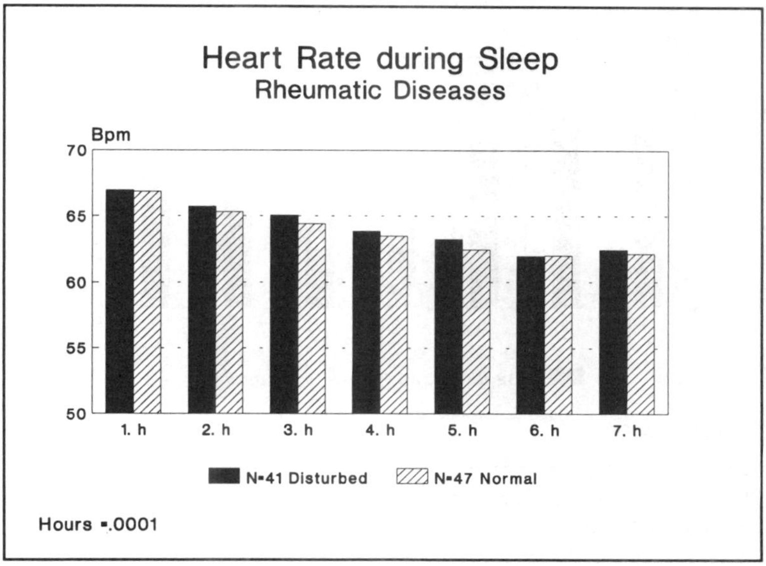

Figure 107. Heart rate during sleep in patients with rheumatic diseases. From Myrtek, 2002, modified. Reproduced with permission. Copyright 2002 by Hogrefe, Göttingen.

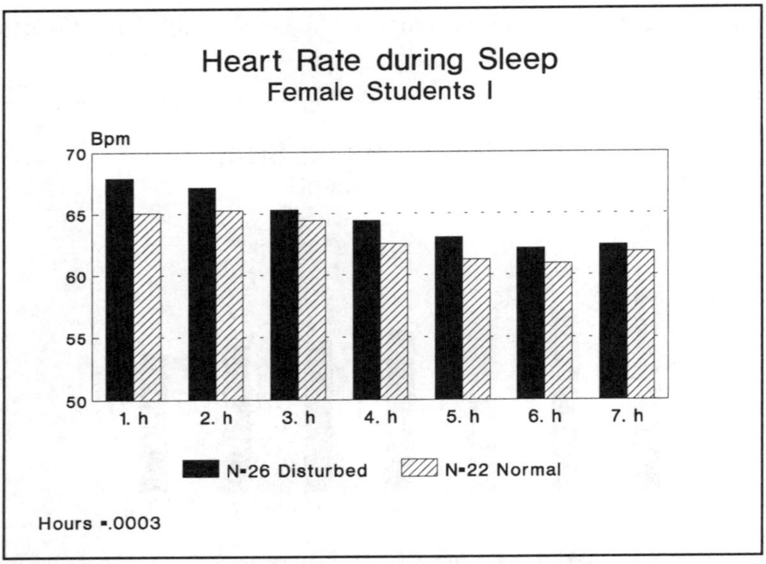

Figure 108. Heart rate during sleep in female students, first sample. From Myrtek, 2002, modified. Reproduced with permission. Copyright 2002 by Hogrefe, Göttingen.

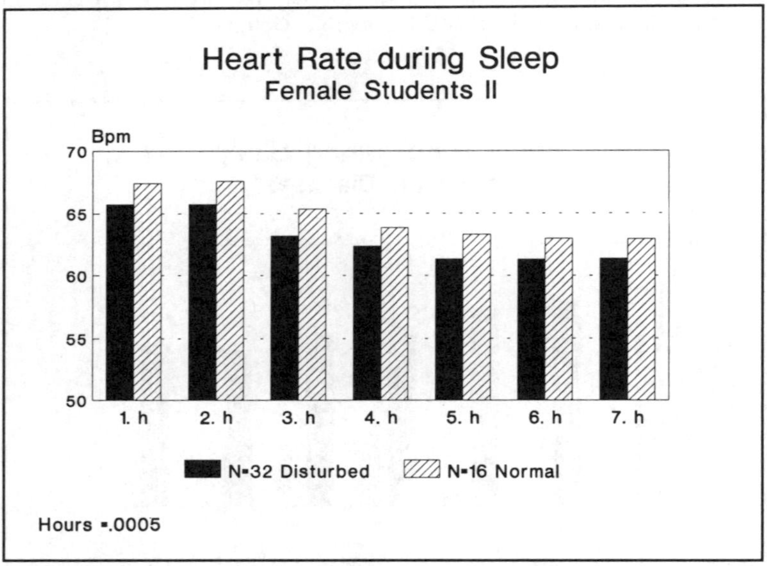

Figure 109. Heart rate during sleep in female students, second sample. From Myrtek, 2002, modified. Reproduced with permission. Copyright 2002 by Hogrefe, Göttingen.

Physical activity (see Figures 110 to 113) was highest in the first hour of the sleeping time in all groups. Presumably, this was caused by going to bed and by finding the right body position for sleep onset. Our hypothesis of a higher physical activity in subjects with sleep disturbances was not substantiated.

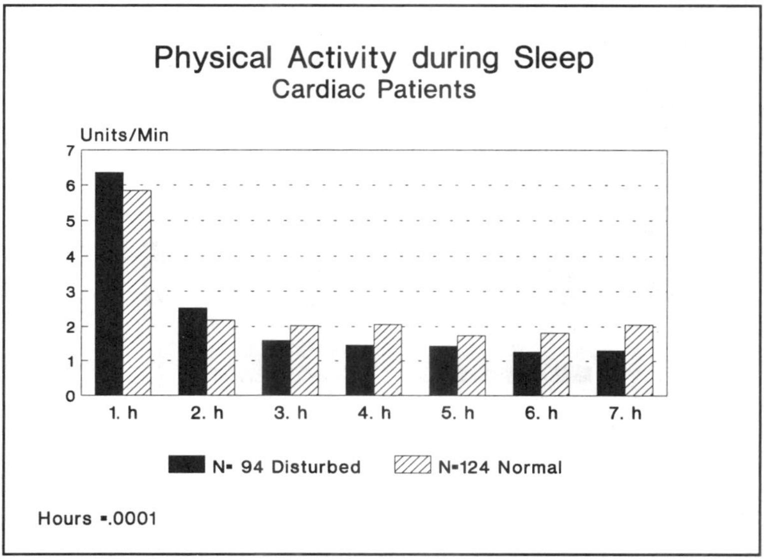

Figure 110. Physical activity during sleep in cardiac patients. From Myrtek, 2002, modified. Reproduced with permission. Copyright 2002 by Hogrefe, Göttingen.

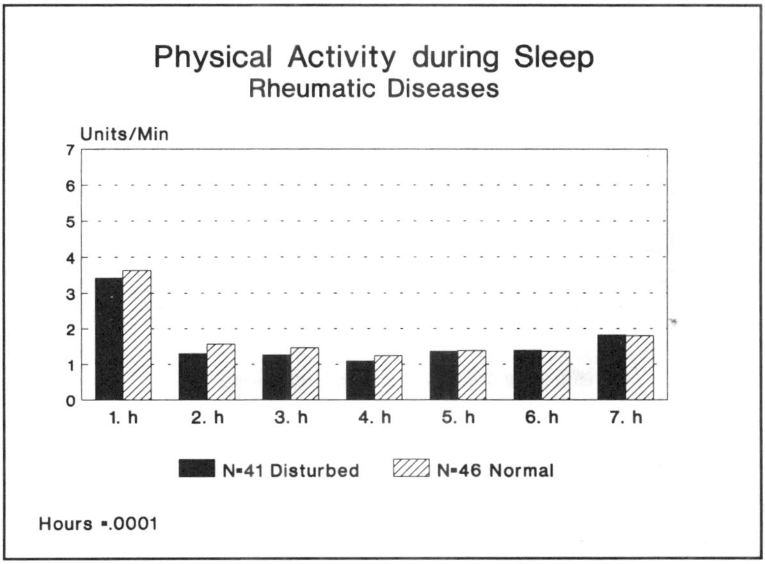

Figure 111. Physical activity during sleep in patients with rheumatic diseases. From Myrtek, 2002, modified. Reproduced with permission. Copyright 2002 by Hogrefe, Göttingen.

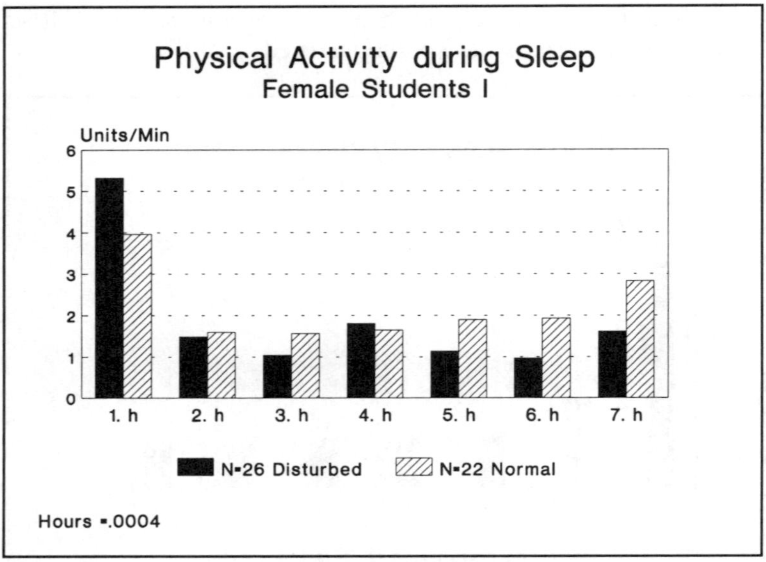

Figure 112. Physical activity during sleep in female students, first sample. From Myrtek, 2002, modified. Reproduced with permission. Copyright 2002 by Hogrefe, Göttingen.

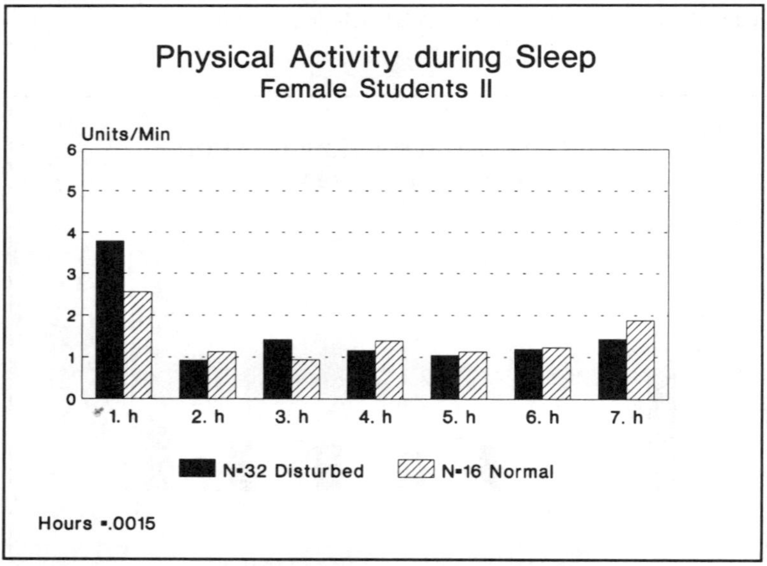

Figure 113. Physical activity during sleep in female students, second sample. From Myrtek, 2002, modified. Reproduced with permission. Copyright 2002 by Hogrefe, Göttingen.

AHR significantly increased during the night and was highest in the seventh hour (see Figures 114 to 117).

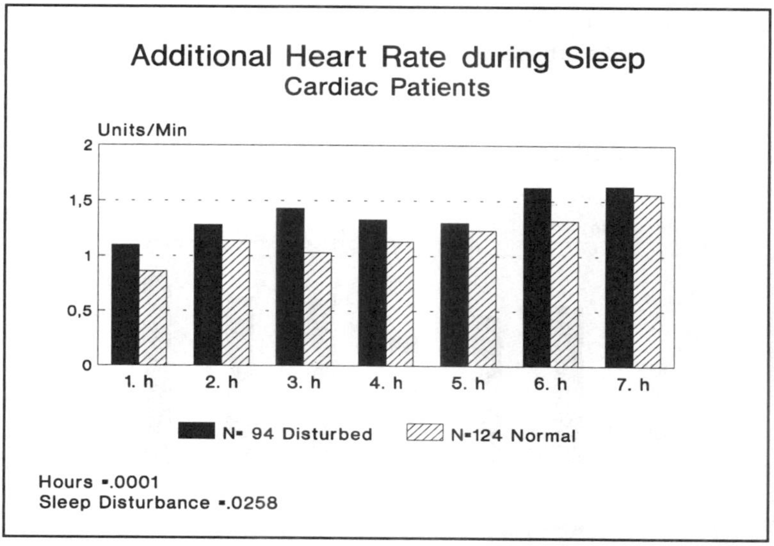

Figure 114. Additional heart rate during sleep in cardiac patients. From Myrtek, 2002, modified. Reproduced with permission. Copyright 2002 by Hogrefe, Göttingen.

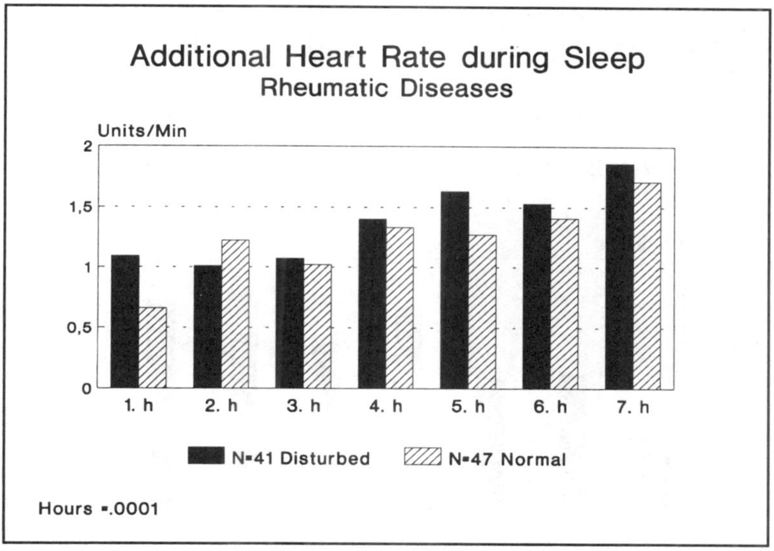

Figure 115. Additional heart rate during sleep in patients with rheumatic diseases. From Myrtek, 2002, modified. Reproduced with permission. Copyright 2002 by Hogrefe, Göttingen.

The hypothesis that AHR might be greater in subjects with sleep disturbances was substantiated in the cardiac patients and in the first student group. In patients with rheumatic diseases, a nearly significant interaction hours * sleep disturbances was observed (p = .079). This means that in the second half of the night AHR increased in patients with sleep disturbances.

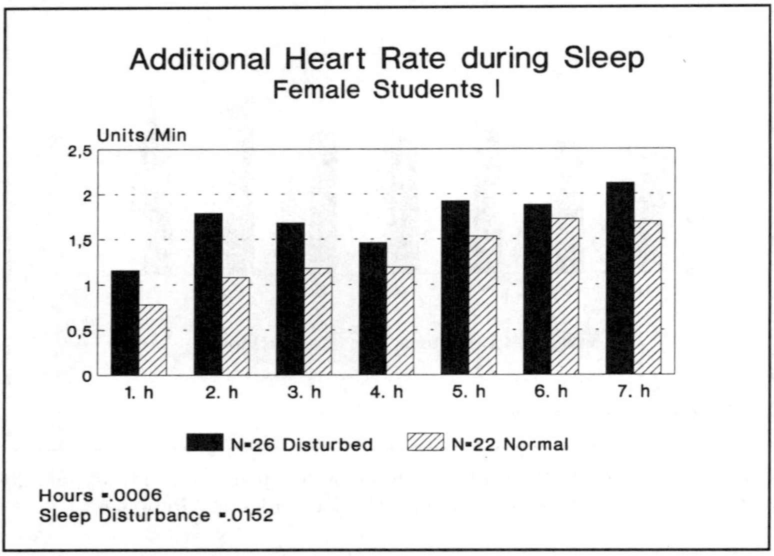

Figure 116. Additional heart rate during sleep in female students, first sample. From Myrtek, 2002, modified. Reproduced with permission. Copyright 2002 by Hogrefe, Göttingen.

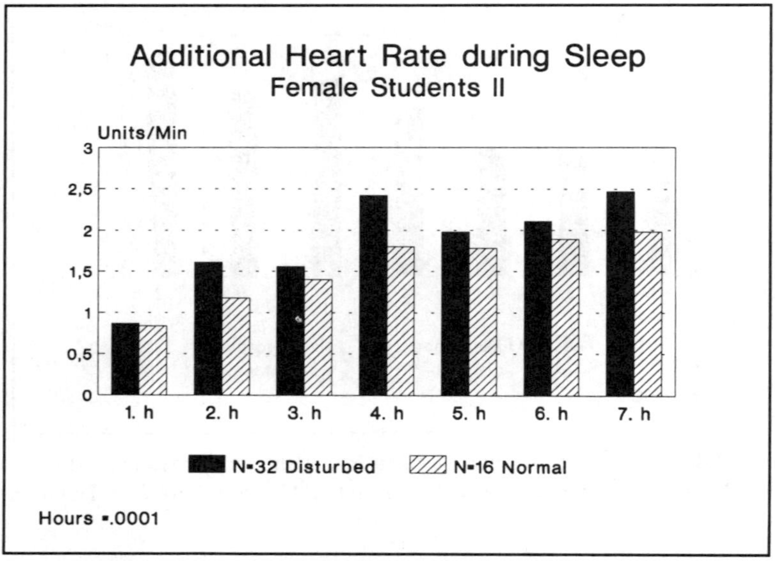

Figure 117. Additional heart rate during sleep in female students, second sample. From Myrtek, 2002, modified. Reproduced with permission. Copyright 2002 by Hogrefe, Göttingen.

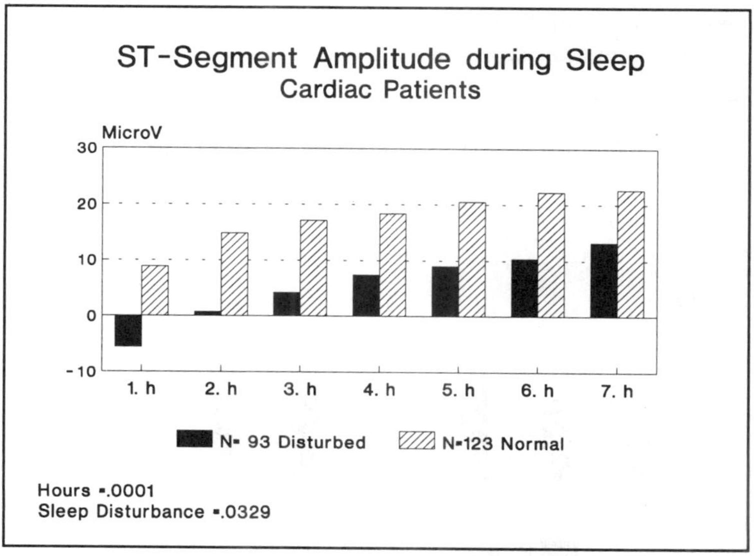

Figure 118. ST-segment amplitude during sleep in cardiac patients From Myrtek, 2002, modified. Reproduced with permission. Copyright 2002 by Hogrefe, Göttingen.

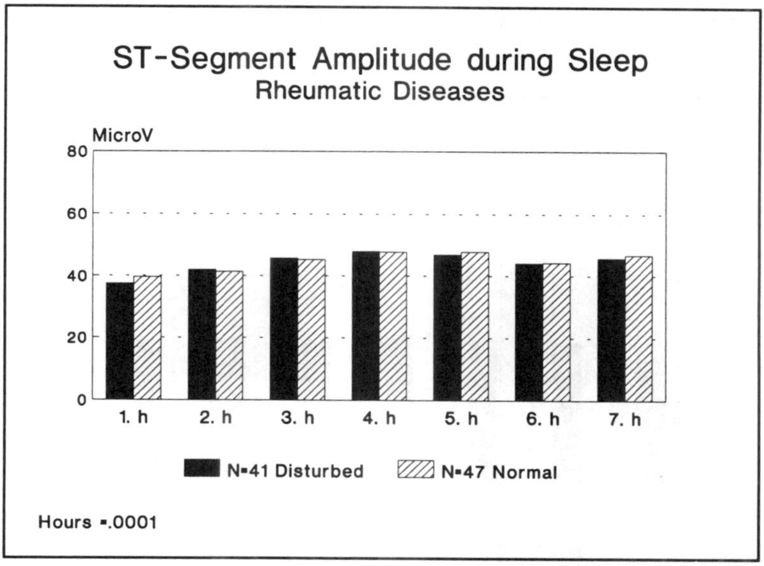

Figure 119. ST-segment amplitude during sleep in patients with rheumatic diseases. From Myrtek, 2002, modified. Reproduced with permission. Copyright 2002 by Hogrefe, Göttingen.

The amplitude of the ST segment significantly increased during the night in three of the groups and was nearly significant in the second student group (p = .063). In cardiac patients and in one of the student groups, subjects with disturbed sleep had lower ST-segment amplitudes (see Figures 118 to121).

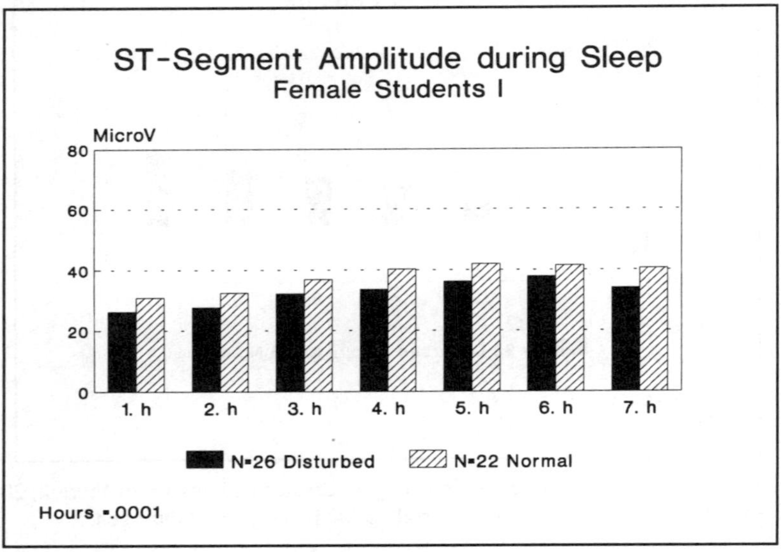

Figure 120. ST-segment amplitude during sleep in female students, first sample. From Myrtek, 2002, modified. Reproduced with permission. Copyright 2002 by Hogrefe, Göttingen.

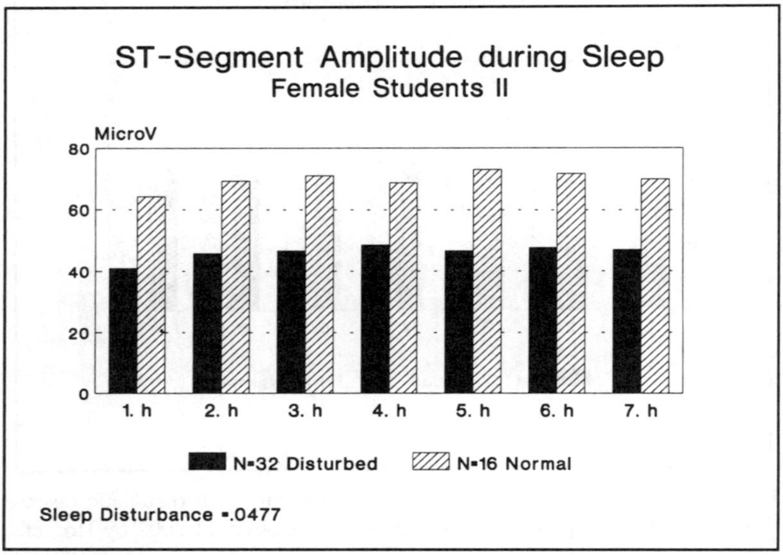

Figure 121. ST-segment amplitude during sleep in female students, second sample. From Myrtek, 2002, modified. Reproduced with permission. Copyright 2002 by Hogrefe, Göttingen.

8.3 Discussion

The hypothesis of a decreasing heart rate during the night was substantiated in all groups. No replicated support was found for a higher heart rate of the sleep disturbed subjects compared to subjects with normal sleep. There was only a tendency for higher heart rate in poor sleepers in the cardiac patient group. It is remarkable that we did not find any differences in physical activity between good and poor sleepers. Most people would hold the opinion that sleep disturbances are accompanied by higher physical activity during night caused by leaving the bed more frequently.

The hypothesis that the increasing duration of REM during the night might lead to an increase of AHR was found in all groups. It is relevant that at least in two samples a significant difference in AHR was found between good and poor sleepers. This means that heart rate fluctuations during the night are more common in poor than in good sleepers. It is noteworthy, however, that these fluctuations are not caused by heart rate variability (MSSD, not displayed in the Figures) because there were no differences between the groups of good and poor sleepers. We can assume that the higher fluctuations in heart rate in poor sleepers are due to a higher sympathetic activity during the night. The higher sympathetic activity is also indicated by the lower ST-segment amplitude in poor sleepers which was found in two samples. It is tempting to speculate about this finding. Possibly, the higher sympathetic activity in subjects with disturbed sleep is accompanied by more dream activity or even nightmares. The psychological findings are in line with this speculation. Emotional lability was higher in all groups. Moreover, the patient groups rated themselves as having physical complaints more frequently and rated more heart pain during the feedbacks. Thus, sleep disturbances are one of the rare examples of a psychophysiological disorder.

8.4 Summary

This Chapter was focused on physiological monitoring with the FMS during sleep. Four of our samples, two patient and two female student samples, were grouped by a simple rating scale in good and poor sleepers. Hypotheses for the course of the physiological parameters were derived from the relevant literature. A continuous decrease in heart during sleep was expected and found in all samples. Not substantiated was the notion of a higher heart rate in poor sleepers. The expectation that poor sleepers are likely to show higher physical activity at night was not found. According to our hypothesis that AHR will increase in the course of the night, an increase was observed in all samples. Interestingly, AHR was higher in poor than in good sleepers in at least two of the samples. We have argued that poor sleepers might have a greater fluctuation in heart rate due to a higher sympathetic activation during sleep. Psychologically, poor sleepers had higher scores in the personality dimension emotional lability. In the patient samples, poor sleepers rated themselves on having physical complaints and heart pain more frequently than good sleepers.

Chapter 9

General discussion

This book deals with the psychophysiological covariation problem, though many people would prefer to see the use of the term mind-body problem. We have already been working on this issue for 35 years. The subject has always been and still is of great interest to many people. Issues such as psychosomatic medicine, alternative medicine, environmental medicine, homeopathic medicine, psychotherapy, and the placebo effect all deal with the covariation problem. I myself, in the early 60's, was deeply impressed by the writings of Freud (1940) and Uexküll (1963). This also influenced the choice of my occupation. Instead of becoming an engineer, I studied medicine and psychology. In 1970, I was given the opportunity to join the Psychophysiological Research Group. This group enabled one to research at a very professional level because the co-workers involved came from quite different disciplines. Moreover, we had sufficient funding to acquire all modern devices.

In the first 10 years, research in the laboratory was done mainly with cardiac patients and students. Important parameters were biochemical measures (e.g., catecholamines, electrolytes), impedance cardiography (e.g., heart rate, cardiac output, ventricular ejection time), blood pressure, pulse wave velocity, electrodermal activity, respiratory parameters (e.g., respiratory minute volume, O_2-uptake, CO_2-output), and anthropometric measures (e.g., skinfold thickness, different circumferences and breadths). The provocation techniques used to alter the activation level of the subjects comprised arithmetic, free speech, reaction time tests, cold pressor test, ergometric exercise on different levels, breath holding, hyperventilation, and orthostatic tests. Needless to say, we also assessed physical complaints, mood, personality dimensions, and anamnestic data. In 1981, a first experiment in a field setting (1000 m run in an athletic stadium) was conducted with a microprocessor-based ambulatory monitoring system (Kunz, Mertens, & Oeste, 1982).

This research was carried out very systematically and resulted in several books and papers: Constitutional psychophysiology (Myrtek, 1984), psychophysiological stress research (Fahrenberg, Walschburger, Foerster, Myrtek, & Müller, 1979; 1983), and laboratory-field studies (Fahrenberg, Foerster, Schneider, Müller, & Myrtek, 1984; 1986). With respect to the covariation problem, first frustrations emerged: "The central finding of the present investigation is the retention of the null hypothesis concerning psychophysiological covariance. This finding is relevant and deserves our attention, since practically all physiological, psychological, and biochemical methods available for this issue at the present time have been thoroughly exhausted on relatively large patient and student samples. The null hypothesis is defined as the lack of correlation between morphological, biochemical, and physiological variables, on the one hand, and psychological variables as assessed by personality questionnaires, state and mood scales, somatic complaint lists, and life habit scales, on the other" (Myrtek, 1984, p. 228).

Obviously, we were not the only ones who observed a lack of psychophysiological covariation. In the manual of the International Classification of Diseases based on the eighth revision conference of the World Health Organization, the three-digit category 305 embraced "Physical disorders of presumably pschogenic origin" (World Health Organization, 1967). In the cardiovascular section, diseases such as "cardiac neurosis" and "neurocirculatory asthenia" were listed. The ninth revision of the ICD listed "306 Physiological malfunction arising from mental factors" (World Health Organization, 1977). The following explanation was given for this category: "A variety of physical symptoms or types of physiological malfunction of mental origin, not involving tissue damage and usually mediated through the autonomic nervous system." In the present tenth revision of the ICD, cardiac neurosis and neurocirculatory asthenia are listed under the "F45 Somatoform disorders", that is, exactly under "F45.3 Somatoform autonomic dysfunction" (World Health Organization, 1992). The following explanation is given: "Symptoms are presented by the patient as if they were due to a physical disorder of a system or organ that is largely or completely under autonomic innervation and control....The symptoms are usually of two types, neither of which indicates a physical disorder of the organ or system concerned. First, there are complaints based upon objective signs of autonomic arousal, such as palpitations, sweating....Second, there are subjective complaints of a nonspecific or changing nature such as fleeting aches and pains, sensations of burning, heaviness,...which are referred by the patient to a specific organ or system" (p. 349).

This development in the ICD revisions surely represents an abandonment of the psychosomatic idea. Our own results, sketched out briefly above, were largely based on laboratory research. This research is viewed to be artificial and of low ecological validity (Fahrenberg, 1996). At least theoretically it might be that psychophysiological observations in the natural environment might lead to another view of the covariation problem. Naturally, ambulatory monitoring studies were feasible to a satisfying degree only in the late 80's because of the technological development.

9.1 Methodological considerations

As already cited in Chapter 1, Cannon (1929) pointed to the "reflex character" of emotional reactions. This means that emotions are very quick. In Chapter 2 we described the baroreceptor reflex. Stimulation of the baroreceptor and onset of vagal bradycardia is about 0.5 s or less. Baroreceptor unloading on the other hand results in tachycardia due to reduced vagal inhibition and increased sympathetic activity. The duration for tachycardia induction is in the same range as for the induction of bradycardia. These quick responses in heart rate are a necessary prerequisite for our method.

The starting point of our method, presented in this book, was the observation that heart rate reactivity elicited by a stressor combination is nearly an additive combination of the respective reactivity elicited by the single stressors. If it would be possible to record the energetical component reliably through the measurement of physical activity, a decomposition of heart rate in the energetical and emotional or mental component would be successful. At first, we thought of a kind of individual calibration through a number of non-emotional standard situations in which both heart rate and physical activity would be measured. Later on under field conditions, when heart rate would be higher than expected from physical activity, we would surmise an emotional event. We early noticed that this method would not work. There are too many situations in everyday life that cannot be included in a set of standard situations. For instance, it would not have been possible to build standard situations for bus or train drivers. So we developed the method with moving averages for both physical activity and heart rate.

With this method, a continuous adaptation to changing physical activity is possible. Because with increasing activity "noise" becomes greater, the amount of heart rate increase for an AHR event increases, too. This begs the question what a minimal heart rate increase in the case of no or only minimal physical activity might actually be. Emotions are mostly short phenomena lasting for only a few seconds. Our unit of analysis is one minute. If we suppose that a given emotion would lead to a heart rate increase of 18 bpm for 10 seconds, this would yield an increase of three bpm for the whole minute. We have chosen this minimal three bpm for the indication of AHR in our algorithm. This decision was based on many empirical tests to determine the range of heart rate and AHR during the development of our method.

The first big advantage of the method is the simplicity of the recording technique. In fact, only heart rate and physical activity are needed. Heart rate is the strongest biosignal of the body in the range of one to three millivolts on the body surface. If the ECG monitoring electrodes are properly attached to the chest using firm points such as sternum and ribs, it is always possible to get a good signal quality. Physical activity presents also no problems. If the accelerative sensors are operating without technical defect, the output does not comprise any artifact. Important is the fact that during monitoring, subjects are not aware of the measurement for most of the time. Compared, e.g., to blood pressure monitoring, no reactivity effects by our method are observed (Shapiro et al., 1996). It is also important that subjects are not hampered by the device as for instance during monitoring of electrodermal activity (EDA) with electrodes on the palms of the hand or the foot. Finally, all our parameters have a wide range of measurement with a good differentiation from baseline to the highest possible activation. When we look, e.g., at EDA, differentiation of activation states stops when the palms are wet. The same is true for an electroencephalogram which only differentiates states of low activation.

A second advantage of our method is the unequivocal interpretation of the parameters. There is no doubt that heart rate represents the total work load component as shown by the many laboratory experiments cited at the beginning of this Chapter. As pointed out in Chapters 1 and 3, physical activity measured at the trunk and the leg really represents physical work load. Naturally, there are several situations in which the notion that physical activity represents the energetical load directly is erroneous. Driving a car produces a physical activity signal of the driver that does not only reflect his energetical load but especially the vibrations of the car. This surely is a disadvantage that has to be accepted. The alternative to wearing a mask in order to determine O_2-consumption has still more disadvantages. We can overcome the difficulties with physical activity to a certain degree if we know what is going on. Through rather frequent feedbacks every 15 minutes, a good deal is known about what subjects are doing. Thus, we can take into account such misinterpretations of physical activity.

The core parameter, however, is AHR. Does AHR really reflect emotional work load? We hope that the reader will be convinced by the many studies conducted for validation (see Chapter 3.4). Naturally, AHR also has limitations. We have already noticed that increases in heart rate due to emotional factors which are accompanied by an increase in physical activity cannot be detected by our method. On the other hand there are certain situations in which AHR is present but not due to emotional factors. We often observed an increase of AHR during the stay at the lavatory. It is known from physiology that, e.g., emptying the bladder is due to a rise in the thoracic and abdominal pressure. By this, heart rate increases which spuriously causes AHR. Another example would be if someone is sitting in the television chair, stands up for a moment to get peanuts from a cupboard, and after that sits down quietly again in the chair. Because the unit of analysis is one minute, physical activity would only minimally increase on average for the whole minute but heart rate increase in this situation would be far more prominent because lifting the body from the chair is relatively strenuous. However, in nearly all other situations an increase of AHR indicates an increase in emotional or mental work load.

Although the interpretation of heart rate, physical activity, and AHR are unequivocal, the use of heart rate variability (MSSD) as an indicator of mental work load is a matter of conjecture. Our studies during work and leisure time have shown that whenever MSSD revealed a significant difference between certain situations, this difference was no longer significant when in the computation heart rate was introduced as a covariate. As we have shown in Chapter 3.4.1, heart rate is negatively correlated with MSSD to a substantial degree. So we have to conclude that MSSD is not a valid indicator of mental work load. We have shown in Chapter 3.5.3 that it makes little sense to differentiate between emotional and mental work load because AHR will be initiated by both loads. We can also assume that emotional and mental work load are mixed in most situations of everyday life.

Besides heart rate variability, we have examined further parameters. In clinical populations it might be worthwhile paying attention to the ST-segment amplitude and ischemic episodes. Because only the first channel of the ECG is optimized for the reliable detection of the R wave for on-line analysis, the second channel can be used for ST-segment analysis. In patients who are known to have ST-segment depression from clinical diagnosis, the electrodes of the second channel can be attached in a way to detect possible ST-segment changes during everyday life. Another parameter we examined was P-wave amplitude. P-wave amplitude increases during both physical activity and emotional work load. This parameter represents sympathetic activation but does not differentiate between physical and emotional work load. Therefore, we have not included P wave in the present descriptions of our studies.

A third advantage of the method is seen in the carefully controlled handling of data. The programs for on-line analysis of heart rate are very robust and reliable. We compared data from on-line analysis with data derived off-line from the ECG and observed nearly no differences. Artifact control was always executed rigorously by a special interactive graphic program. Mostly, however, it was not necessary to eliminate any data from the record except when an electrode had become detached. Of importance are the many but short feedbacks during monitoring which are emitted on average every 15 minutes. This enables one to get a detailed protocol throughout the day. With a special program, we can work down this protocol through the data and can do a plausibility control. Segmentation of the whole record with the behavioral data derived from the feedbacks is done in fine detail. This enables a time-locked analysis of behavior, subjective state, and work load components.

9.2 Interoception and emotions

With our method it is possible to examine the question, to what extent are emotions and physical complaints based on interoception. Undoubtedly, true feedbacks which are based on AHR are accompanied by a heart rate increase. In case of interoception we would, therefore, expect a significant difference in the subjective state between true and random feedback. At least ratings of excitement performed during feedback should be higher during true than during random feedback. Our studies have shown, however, that healthy subjects as well as patients with cardiovascular diseases or cardiac neurosis were not able to discern these different physiological states correctly.

This means that the ratings of excitement are obviously not based on interoception but are determined by other mechanisms. Pennebaker (1982) observed that reported physical symptoms were inversely related to the amount of external information determined by situational circumstances. There is a "competition of cues" between the internal and external information with more external cues mitigating the perception of the internal cues. Pennebaker reported that his jogging time on a cross-country track was faster than on a standard circular lap track of comparable distance. Moreover, fatigue on the lap track was higher than on the cross-country course. The explanation was that the lap track requires minimal processing of external information as compared to the cross-country track. Therefore, the probability of noticing physical sensations on the lap track is greater than on the cross-country course. In Pennebaker's jogging study with students over two weeks, jogging time was consistently lower on the cross-country track than on the lap track. The reported level of fatigue, however, was the same on both tracks.

The competition of cues hypothesis surely might partly explain the findings for true and random feedbacks. In everyday life there are a lot of competing external cues. However, even more important for the explanation of our findings might be the hypothesis of cognitive schemas. The students in our laboratory experiment with erotic and pornographic movies rated the latter to be more exciting than the former although the physiological parameters revealed just the opposite. Clearly, cognitive schemas concerning the arousal potential of erotic movies are involved.

Cognitive schemas based on psychological factors also form the interpretative basis for our study with asymptomatic (AMI) and symptomatic myocardial (SMI) patients (see Chapter 4.3.2). SMI patients revealed more emotional lability, less health satisfaction, and rated more frequently as having physical complaints than the AMI patients, although no differences in the medical parameters were observed. On the contrary, AMI patients showed more premature contractions. During monitoring, SMI patients rated as being more excited, experiencing less enjoyment, and having more heart pain than AMI patients. A consequence of this study is the notion that angina pectoris is no secure indicator for an underlying CHD. This notion was also confirmed in the study on emotional arousal and ischemic episodes in CHD patients (see Chapter 4.3.4). The comparison of ischemic episodes with control episodes showed no difference in anginal pain.

A sufficient interoception of physiological functions is the prerequisite for the *medical model* as already stated in Chapter 4.4. This model is based on the assumption that physical complaints have an underlying physiological reason. This might be true for acute diseases such as an appendicitis. Our findings with chronic diseases, however, reveal that this model does not work. A chronic organic impairment will or will not be accompanied by physical complaints and healthy persons will or will not complain about physical symptoms. This also means that there is no firm association between physical complaints and the severeness of a disease (Myrtek, 2001). We have called the phenomena of physical complaints without impairment and of impairment without complaints *inadequate illness behavior*. Obviously, there is a striking difference between *illness* and *disease* (Barondess, 1979; Dworkin, 1991; Ford, 1983). Illness represents in the English language the subjective state with physical complaints and disease actually is based on an organic impairment. In the German language we do not draw such a distinction.

The health care systems – be it in the Anglo-American countries or in Germany – are based, on the assumption that the medical model is correct. This, however, has serious consequences for all people. When we state that chronic diseases are not accompanied by physical complaints in all cases, then only a systematic screening method would be adequate to check the state of health in the population. Such screening methods, however, are the exception from the rule. Medical examinations of 595 persons in the USA by Coulehan (1975) revealed that 11% had diseases which should be treated such as diseases of the kidneys, the liver, hypertension, diabetes, etc. In another 7% diseases were known but these were not under medical treatment. In Germany, 2,429 workers aged more than 40 years were medically screened for frequent diseases (Böck, Rommel, & Schröder, 1979; Rommel, Steinhardt, & Überla, 1976). Of these workers, 1,192 persons had at least one pathological finding such as hypercholesteremia, hypertension, heart disease, etc. In medical examinations with 15,193 men aged 40 to 49 years working in two big companies, physicians advised 0.6% of the workers to be treated in a hospital (Robra, van der Heyden, & Machens, 1982). Given these facts we must state that the health care systems are not working optimally. The first diagnosis of a disease is made either by a medical laymen, the prospective patient, or by his unprofessional social environment. So we have a situation in which many persons being treated in the health care systems who are not medically diseased, whereas other persons are active at the workplace with serious diseases.

The opinion that emotions are based on interoception is widely held. Therefore, we might expect differences in the frequency of emotions reported between true and random feedback. However, only for anxiety/fear a significant difference was observed in our student samples. This means that the report of an emotion in everyday life is often not based on interoception. It also seems that report of emotion is dependent upon the situational circumstances because reports were more frequent during interactions with friends compared to interactions with other students.

Especially relevant for the issue of emotion are again cognitive schemas. It was shown that our student groups held the same view in the subjective description of the different emotions we asked for. We can assume that everybody in his life has perceived emotions such as anxiety, anger, and happiness. However, such states are rather rare events. As proposed by Rimé et al. (1990), these experiences might form emotional prototypes which are evoked in situations with emotional cues. This might also explain the lack of a physiological differentiation we found for the different emotions. However, still another explanation for the absence of physiological profiles might be true. As Gray (1994) pointed out, all emotions require energy mobilization which might not lead to special profiles for different emotions.

Especially interesting was the result concerning the accuracy of emotion perception. The percentage of correctly classified true feedbacks (emotion present) was negatively correlated to a high degree with the percentage of correctly classified random feedbacks (no emotion present) in all samples. It seems that two subject groups are present in our samples, one group who often report emotions and another group reporting emotions less frequently. In case of the first group, a higher percentage of correct classified true feedbacks and a lower percentage of correct classified random feedbacks are to be expected and in the second group the reverse. This finding clearly represents a cognitive schema, too. Regardless of the different physiological arousal in true and random feedback, "emotional subjects" frequently report emotions whereas "cool subjects" seldom report emotions.

Our studies on emotions are the first ones which did not rely on self-reported emotions but on emotionally-induced physiological activation. In this way it is possible to answer the question, to what extent physiological activation of emotional origin is perceived. We have to state that strong emotional arousal which can be easily perceived is obviously a rare event in everyday life. This follows from the fact that the percentage of emotions reported for true and random feedback was not significantly different, with the exception of anxiety. Nevertheless, subjects reported on emotions to a considerable degree. Female students rated about 40% of the feedbacks to be of emotional origin whereas male students identified about 30%, the sex difference being significant. These high percentages are surely also caused by the fact that the students knew they were taking part in a field experiment to study emotions. If one would ask students how frequently they perceive an emotion on a normal day, the figure would be considerably smaller. Taken all together, emotion report in everyday life can be based on interoception but mostly is inferred from situational circumstances and cognitive schemas.

9.3 Stress and strain

Since the popular writings by Selye (1950, 1956), stress is the most popular concept for psychologists and for laymen. In a representative population survey with 2,035 persons, 52% of all people aged 16 to 80 agreed to the statement "I often have stress" (Fahrenberg et al., 1984). During their stay at a health resort, 87 myocardial infarction patients were asked to disclose their opinion concerning the causes of their infarction. Stress at work and time pressure scaled highest, whereas classical risk factors such as smoking, hypertension, and blood lipids were rated to be low or medium (Fahrenberg, Myrtek, & Trichtinger, 1985). This finding was confirmed in another study with 124 coronary patients (Kreutel, 1989). However, the notion that subjective stress might be an independent risk factor of CHD is not proven (Myrtek, 1997, 1998a).

9.3.1 Stress at the workplace

Ambulatory monitoring studies at the workplace are rare and studies which have tried to evaluate special aspects of the work, as done with the studies in drivers and dispatchers, are nonexistent (see Chapter 6). Insofar, these studies are unique. The most important result of all our studies is the fact that neither the subjective evaluation of the work load nor the objective evaluation by the observers was consistent with the physiological work load components, especially with the emotional component. This means that the real strain of a work imposed on a person cannot be inferred from any subjective or objective stress rating.

However, subjective stress ratings concerning work load are important for other reasons. Bigos and coworkers (1991) conducted a prospective study with 3,020 aircraft employees to identify risk factors for reported acute back pain at work. After four years of follow-up, 279 subjects reported back pain. Subjects who did not enjoy their work were 2.5 times more likely to report back pain than subjects who enjoyed it. This study already reveals that a correlation exists between subjective stress ratings and physical complaints. Watson and Pennebaker (1989) investigated 164 students. The subjective stress ratings correlated significantly with several health complaint scales (0.31 to 0.36). In a study with 328 train drivers who encountered fatal or near fatal accidents (Myrtek, Itte, Zimmermann, & Brügner, 1994), stress was assessed according to DSM-III-R criteria for the diagnosis of Posttraumatic Stress Disorder (PTSD) on a five-point scale. The PTSD-scale correlated 0.36 with physical complaints and 0.16 ($p = .003$) with FLZ work satisfaction. This means that train drivers who had higher ratings for stress had also more physical complaints and were more dissatisfied with their work. After the accident, drivers who scored low on the PTSD-scale were on average 2.9 days on sick-leave and high scorers 11.1 days. Subjective stress ratings are clearly important for health care systems and for economic reasons but do not necessarily reflect work load.

In train drivers, the driving modes "start" and "braking to halt" were especially strenuous. The instructors or the drivers themselves did not know this before this study. Both groups were convinced that other modes of driving, especially braking on the mountain track, would imply high emotional work load. However, as our results have shown, this mode was emotionally with little effect. Different train speeds up to 100 km/h were not important factors for work load, and higher speeds up to 200 km/h showed a monotony effect with decreasing heart rate the higher the speed. The latter was clearly due to a tunnel effect caused by the electric poles.

With increasing number of braking operations, the bus drivers' heart rate increased. This was at least partly due to an increase in physical activity. The observer ratings but not the self ratings were in accordance with the physiological findings. We thought that increasing traffic density, rated on a three-step scale by the observers, might be a source of stress and work load (not described in Chapter 6.1). However, work load components were not different for the high traffic situations. Only the ratings made by the observers were compatible with our assumption. As in the train drivers, heart rate and AHR were higher during starting than during movement at various speeds of the bus. Heart rate also decreased with increasing speed.

For dispatchers, total work load was dependent on the number of trains they had to manage at the same time but AHR was not significantly different. The ratings of both observers and dispatchers were in accordance with total work load. Total work load was especially high during special train services. But these situations were rare and were not included in our results.

In Chapter 6.2, work load components in white and blue collar workers during a normal shift at an industrial plant were examined. Higher heart rate and higher physical activity was expected for the blue collar workers than for the white collar workers. These differences were observed but no difference for AHR emerged. The latter finding contradicts the view that white collar workers are subjected to higher mental or emotional work load. During the working hours heart rate, physical activity, and AHR showed different profiles but we cannot interpret these differences because we did not ask about associated special activities during work. In contrast to the other hours, lunch break values between 12.00 and 13.00 h were prominent. Physical activity and heart rate were lower but AHR showed a peak. We assume that this finding was caused by social contact with other employees. Contrary to the physiological findings, ratings of excitement and enjoyment differentiated neither the worker groups nor the hours during the shift.

In the first study with university students (see Chapter 6.3), heart rate was actually higher while staying at the university than being at home, with no differences in physical activity. AHR was also higher at the university but was significant only for the male students. In accordance with these findings, higher excitement and less enjoyment was rated at the university compared to home. But the second study with university students failed to replicate the finding for AHR.

During classroom tests as compared to normal lessons in schoolboys, heart rate was higher during the tests (see Chapter 6.4). Interestingly, the older boys showed higher heart rate reactivity than the younger boys during both tests and normal lessons. The older boys also revealed a tendency to react higher even during the tests. The same pattern was observed for the subjective ratings of excitement and enjoyment. Older boys rated more excitement and less enjoyment during the tests. These findings may be interpreted such that tests are far more important for the older than for the younger boys.

9.3.2 Stress during leisure time

The most surprising result in train and bus drivers as well as dispatchers was that AHR was higher in all groups during leisure time than during work (see Chapter 7.1). This is contrary to the notion held by most people. Our result concerning AHR was confirmed by the white and blue collar workers, too (see Chapter 7.2). We have to state that emotional work load is higher during leisure time than during work. Contrary to this physiological finding are the subjective ratings of the white and blue collar workers. Leisure time was rated as less exciting and more enjoyable than working time. Clearly, these ratings are not based on interoceptions but on cognitive schemas.

This notion is further confirmed by our findings in schoolboys (see Chapter 7.3). AHR was consistently higher during TV viewing than during school time. At school, however, excitement was rated as higher and enjoyment as lower. Of importance is the observation that emotional reactivity is dependent on the amount of TV viewing. We have already discussed the possible implication of this finding in detail (see Chapter 7.6).

Indeed, the results of our driving studies are in line with this finding of a discrepancy between physiological reactivity and ratings of the subjective state during work and leisure time (see Chapter 7.4). Emotional work load in our industrial workers was much higher during active driving than during either work or leisure time. However, this was not mirrored by the ratings of subjective state. These results were confirmed by the students driving a car to an amusement park. Emotional work load during the drive was high but excitement and enjoyment were rated as high as in other normal situations during the day.

That certain attractions at the amusement park would indicate high stress situations was expected. The most extreme attraction was the swingboat, increasing basal heart rate more than 50 bpm. According to this, AHR was also extremely high. This is surely an emergency reaction as described by Cannon (1929; see Chapter 1.2.2). This poses the question, why people seek amusement with such attractions. According to Apter (1992), arousing situations are evaluated differently. If the arousal increases within the so-called "protective frame" excitement is experienced to be positive, outside this frame growing excitement evokes anxiety. Obviously, this is a matter of psychology because the physiological reactions on the swing board and also on the roller coaster clearly show an emergency reaction.

9.4 Monitoring during sleep

Heart rate decreased in all of our samples during the night (see Chapter 8). This is an indication of reduced sympathetic and higher parasympathetic activity. The increase of the ST-segment amplitude during the night points in the same direction. An increase of the ST-segment amplitude was also observed in a former study with 31 cardiac patients (Myrtek, Brügner, & Fichtler, 1990). Moreover it is known that myocardial infarction, sudden cardiac death, and myocardial ischemia are less frequent at night. The peak for these cardiac events is in the morning between 6.00 and 12.00 h (Kraft & Martin, 1995).

In all samples, AHR increased during the night. This was obviously due to an increasing REM duration in the course of the night. Interestingly, AHR was higher in poor than in good sleepers, indicating more heart rate fluctuations during sleep in poor sleepers. Because no differences between good and poor sleepers were found in heart rate variability, the finding of more heart rate fluctuations in poor sleepers was attributed to a higher sympathetic activity. In a study by Martinez-Lavin et al. (1998), too, no differences for heart rate variability were found in good and poor sleepers.

An alternative explanation for the heart rate fluctuations would be that parasympathetic activity is decreased in poor sleepers. However, this explanation is not very likely because in this case differences in MSSD had to be observed. As shown by Fahrenberg and Foerster (1991), a very high correlation of $r = 0.91$ exists between MSSD and respiratory sinus arrhythmia (RSA). RSA on the other hand is an indicator of the parasympathetic activity of the heart (Berntson et al., 1994; Cacioppo et al., 1994). Otzenberger and co-workers (1998) investigated the relation between MSSD and the high frequency component of the RR interval in 15 adults. The intraindividual correlations ranged from $r = 0.88$ to $r = 0.97$. Therefore, we can assume that the higher fluctuations in heart rate in poor sleepers are due to a higher sympathetic activity during the night.

9.5 Conclusions

Evolution has developed emotional reactions which are very quick and adaptive. Many thousands of years ago man could only survive dangerous situations by fight or flight. The prerequisite for these activities was a quick increase in cardiac output to enable the necessary blood supply to the muscles. The most important factor for the increase in cardiac output is heart rate. Tachycardia can be evoked within less than one second. This reflex is the basis of our ambulatory monitoring in everyday life. As shown in the present book, the method is feasible and was successfully applied to more than 1,300 subjects of different age groups and different occupations. The method was used for different research questions such as interoception, perception of emotions as well as stress at work and during leisure time. The main results are:

- Interoception hardly or indeed does not take place;
- The perception of emotions in everyday life is mostly based on situational circumstances and cognitive schemas;
- Subjective ratings of stress at work and even observer ratings do not mirror the real work load; and
- Leisure time often is more stressful than work itself.

As we have pointed out, insufficient perception is not a sound basis for the medical model. This model works in the presence of acute diseases but does not work in chronic diseases. Merely failing to perceive physical complaints is no guarantee that a person is healthy. The only way to determine the state of health is a medical examination. Therefore, only medical screenings for chronic diseases on a regular basis would be able to detect diseases at their onset. Such screening is offered by the health system for special diseases and for special age groups such as cancer of the breast and the prostate. However, the utilization of these services depends on the individual, although most people do not make use of screening examinations. There are of course many people in the medical health care system who are not physically ill but perceive physical symptoms. Somatization is a very frequent phenomenon. Indeed, 10% to 30% of all patients present bodily complaints to primary care physicians for which no physical cause is subsequently detected (Kellner, 1991). According to Ketterer and Buckholtz (1989), the most serious complications are iatrogenic such as abuse of psychoactive substances or unnecessary surgery. For these patients only a psychological treatment would be adequate.

The issue of emotion perception has less serious consequences than those stated for the perception of physical complaints. As pointed out, strong affective states with behavioral responses and physiological activations seem to be rare in everyday life. Therefore, our findings on emotion perception are essentially of theoretical importance. The lack of AHR perception surely has an advantage, too. AHR during the day is rather frequent as stated in Chapter 3.5.1. To perceive all of these events would severely disturb the activities of daily life. So it is economic to perceive only the most prominent AHR events. Of psychological interest is the fact that subjects have different opinions about their emotional reactivity. The notion of emotional and cool subjects is a good example of cognitive schemas. These schemas are independent of the individual number of AHR events.

Of great importance is the fact that the subjective stress ratings at work are not correlated with the real work load components. Work psychology and even work medicine are nearly always based on subjective reports and on reports made by observers. It is not possible to assess strain at work by such reports without physiological monitoring. Stress and life event research based on subjective reports (e.g., Rahe, 1974; Theorell, Lind, & Floderus, 1975) was not very successful and was heavily criticized (e.g., Jenkins, 1976). A more recent large-scale prospective study with 12,866 men also found no correlation between life events and CHD mortality or myocardial infarction (Hollis, Connett, Stevens, & Greenlick, 1990). According to Cannon (1929), an emergency reaction that is not worked off might have pathological effects. Nowadays it is not possible to work off emotional activation as done thousands years ago. So we have to assume that high levels of emotional work load bear a risk for our health.

In an own study it was shown that AHR was accompanied by ischemic episodes in CHD patients (Myrtek et al., 2000). In a small study with three patients who had an implanted cardioverter defibrillator, the causes for a ventricular tachycardia were analyzed (Hofmann et al., 1999). There was a relation between arrhythmia-onset and emotional stress such as public speaking, panic-attack-like anticipation of an unfavorable outcome, and anger reaction superimposed on feelings of helplessness. Leor, Poole, and Kloner (1996) analyzed the relation between an earthquake that struck the Los Angeles area and sudden cardiac death. On the day of the earthquake, there was a sharp increase in the number of sudden deaths from cardiac causes, that is, from a daily average of 4.6 in the preceding week to 24 on the day of the earthquake. All these results suggests that emotional stress may precipitate cardiac events at least in people who are predisposed to such events.

We were rather surprised to establish that leisure time was more stressful than working time, as indicated by AHR. This finding was observed in quite different samples such as train drivers, blue and white collar workers, etc. This is in contrast to the opinion people commonly hold that leisure time is relaxing and a time of recreation. Our subjects also shared this opinion; they rated leisure time to be less exciting and more enjoyable than working time. Comparable results were found in our schoolboy samples. TV viewing revealed higher emotional load than staying at school but subjective stress was rated to exist at school and not during TV viewing. We were also impressed by the high emotional load caused by driving a car. If emotional stress is a risk factor for CHD, and we are convinced that it is, then driving a car is twice as dangerous, first, because of possible accidents, and second, as a risk factor for chronic diseases. Hitherto, this second aspect has not been recognized. On the contrary, people think driving is far more relaxing than staying at work.

At the beginning of this Chapter we have posed the question whether the lack of covariation between physiological parameters and ratings of the subjective state observed in the laboratory might be different in observations made in everyday life. As we have shown, our ecologically valid monitoring lends clear support to the laboratory findings. Psychological parameters are governed by cognitive schemas and are not derived from interoception. The exception to this rule are acute affective states such as anxiety, but such states are rare in healthy subjects. Our findings are especially important because all results have been replicated. The recognition of these findings should have serious consequences for psychological theories such as these pertaining to emotion and stress and for illness and disease in the health care systems. Ambulatory monitoring has also led to new insights, especially through our studies on work and leisure time. We hope that in the future this method will offer quite new perspectives for research in psychology and medicine.

Summary

Emotional reactions are very quick and subserve adaptive mechanisms for survival through flight or fight. Most important for flight or fight is an increase in cardiac output in order to adequately supply the muscles with oxygen. Essentially, cardiac output increase is realized by an increase in heart rate. Heart rate increase will therefore be observed in emotional situations *and* during physical activity, as everybody knows. The Freiburg Monitoring System (FMS) is based on this observation and relies on the decomposition of heart rate in a physical or energetical and in an emotional or psychological component. The physical component of heart rate is assessed by physical activity using a system of accelerative sensors attached on the trunk and the leg. Heart rate is measured by the electrocardiogram (ECG) with electrodes placed on the chest. Both heart rate and physical activity are compared on-line with the help of a minicomputer on a one minute basis. If heart rate of a given minute exceeds the rate of the previous minutes (moving average of three minutes) to a substantial degree without an accompanying increase of physical activity, an emotional event (additional heart rate, AHR) may be assumed. In such a case, the subject is requested by a beep signal to answer relevant questions, given on the display of the device, on how he or she feels, about what he or she is doing, etc. These feedbacks induced by AHR are called "true feedbacks". For reasons of comparison, so-called "random feedbacks" are interspersed and which do not indicate an emotional event. On average, four feedbacks are given per hour.

The validity of the method was assessed in several studies comprising white and blue collar workers, train and bus drivers, railway dispatchers, schoolboys, female students, and male students. Laboratory experiments, in which emotional arousal was induced by movies, served to further validate the AHR. From these studies it was concluded that heart rate is an indicator of total work load, physical activity an indicator of the physical work load component, heart rate variability (mean squared successive differences of the ECG R wave, MSSD) an indicator of the mental, and AHR an indicator of the emotional work load component.

The first issue to be dealt with was interoception, this means the perception of bodily sensations such as palpitations of the heart and chest pain. Interoception is crucial for the *medical model* used in health care systems. This model suggests that a person will be regarded as healthy when physical complaints are absent. The model works well under conditions of acute impairment but is not suitable in chronic diseases. The many sensors inside the body (mechanical, chemical) serve autonomic control but do not inform about the state of the body correctly. Therefore, the information from inside the body is equivocal and open for interpretation. The interpretation is dependant on situational factors, cognitive schemas, personality traits, etc.

Comparisons of true feedbacks with random feedbacks in studies with healthy persons and patients with coronary heart disease (CHD) have shown that subjects were not able to discern these different situations. This means that heart rate cannot be perceived properly. Laboratory studies with students revealed that interoception was dependent on cognitive schemas. Subjects rated, e.g., the pornographic part of a movie as more exciting than the erotic part, although AHR and heart rate were significantly higher during the erotic part.

An important finding in CHD patients was that the perception of heart pain was not dependent on the physiological state of the heart. The comparison of ischemic episodes (depression of the ST segment in the ECG) with control episodes in patients with CHD showed no difference in anginal pain. This means that the absence of angina pectoris is no indicator for the absence of a CHD. With medical examinations only, a CHD can be ruled out. It was also shown that AHR is associated with ST-segment depression. This means that emotional arousal might have adverse effects on the heart.

A second issue pertained to the perception of emotions in everyday life concerns the following. With each feedback, three student samples were asked to disclose possible emotions they perceived. The following emotions were listed on the display of the device: happiness, anger, anxiety/fear, sadness, surprise, disgust, and no emotion. Female students reported in about 40% and male students in about 30% of all feedbacks an emotion. The most frequent emotion was happiness followed by anger and anxiety/fear. All other emotions were rare. Subjectively, anger and anxiety/fear were significantly more exciting and less enjoyable than happiness but no differences between anger and anxiety/fear were observed. Both sexes rated the subjective quality of the emotions very similarly.

If we assume that emotions are based on interoception, we would expect differences in the frequency of emotions reported during true and random feedback. However, only for anxiety/fear was a significant difference observed. It seems that in everyday life strong emotions are rare and emotion reports are mainly based on situational circumstances and not on perception. This might also explain why reproducible physiological profiles for the differing emotions could not be found. The result also revealed that some subjects often reported emotions for both true and random feedback, whereas other subjects did not. Obviously, these differences are based on cognitive schemas. Finally, for anxiety/fear reproducible correlations with personality dimensions such as emotional lability were observed.

The third issue was dealt with stress and strain during work and leisure time. Train and bus drivers as well as dispatchers were accompanied by two observers who rated special work tasks and the amount of stress imposed on the subjects for each minute of the observation. Subjects themselves rated stress every five minutes. The most important result was that both stress ratings often did show no relation with the physiological work load indicators. A study of white and blue collar workers during a normal shift revealed more physical work load for the latter but no difference in emotional work load as indicated by AHR.

Two studies with female and male university students showed that heart rate was higher when staying at the university than being at home. Excitement was rated as greater at the university whereas enjoyment was rated as higher at home. In a study with schoolboys, classroom tests were compared to normal lessons. Total work load as indicated by heart rate was higher during classroom tests. As could be expected, excitement was higher during the tests and enjoyment was lower.

During leisure time, AHR was higher than during work in train drivers, bus drivers, and dispatchers. This result was replicated by the findings made in the blue and white collar workers. However, leisure time was rated as more enjoyable and less exciting than staying at work in all groups. In the studies with schoolboys, TV viewing in the home environment was compared to school time. TV viewing was emotionally far more stressful than school time as indicated by AHR. Again, staying at school was rated as more exciting and less pleasant than viewing TV. An important result was that AHR depends on the amount of TV consumption. Boys with heavy TV consumption showed lower AHR compared to boys with light consumption. The same was true for older as compared to younger boys. This finding was interpreted as emotional bluntness presumably caused by the amount of TV consumption.

Driving a car is very common in everyday life and largely viewed as not being especially stressful. However, AHR was much greater during driving than during working hours in blue and white collar workers. The result was replicated in students driving to an amusement park. Both groups did not perceive the high emotional load because excitement or enjoyment were not rated differently compared to the working hours in blue and white collar workers or to the total daytime in students. A last example of stress during leisure time was given in relation to attractions at an amusement park. Students' heart rate and AHR were extremely high during both the ride on a roller coaster and on a big swingboat. Here, too, subjective ratings of excitement correlated only partly with the physiological reactions.

The final issue dealt with physiological monitoring during sleep. According to hypotheses derived from the literature, a continuous decrease in heart and an increase of AHR due to the rapid eye movement sleep was expected during the course of the night. These hypotheses were substantiated in all four samples. Moreover, each sample was grouped into good and poor sleepers according to a rating scale for sleep disturbances. The expectation that poor sleepers are likely to show higher physical activity at night was not verified. However, in two samples AHR was higher in poor than in good sleepers, this presumably due to greater fluctuations in heart rate caused by higher sympathetic activation during sleep. Psychologically, poor sleepers had higher scores in the personality dimension of emotional lability. In the patient samples, poor sleepers reported physical complaints and heart pain more frequently than good sleepers.

The results of the many studies were discussed within the context of the psychophysiological covariation problem. All findings converge in support of the notion that subjective ratings of the physical state (stress, physical complaints, etc.) are not correlated with the physiological findings. The multiple replication of this fact in healthy subjects and patients during monitoring in real life should have consequences for psychology and medicine.

References

Ambepityia, G., Kopelman, P.G., Ingram, D., Swash, M., Mills, P.G. & Timmis, A.D. (1990). Exertional myocardial ischemia in diabetes: a quantitative analysis of anginal perceptual threshold and the influence of autonomic function. *Journal of the American College of Cardiology*, *15*, 72–77.

Anderson, T.W. (1984). *Introduction to multivariate statistical analysis* (pp. 164–167). New York: John Wiley & Sons.

Antoni, H. (1997). Erregungsphysiologie des Herzens. In: R.F. Schmidt & G. Thews (Eds.), *Physiologie des Menschen*, 27th edition (pp. 472–497). Berlin: Springer.

Apter, M.J. (1992). The dangerous edge. The psychology of excitement. New York: Free Press.

Aureli, F., Preston, S.D. & de Waal, F.B. (1999). Heart rate responses to social interactions in free-moving rhesus macaques (Macaca mulatta): a pilot study. *Journal of Comparative Psychology*, *113*, 59–65.

Averill, J.R., Opton, E.M. & Lazarus, R.S. (1971). Cross-cultural studies of psychophysiological responses during stress and emotion. In: L. Levi (Ed.), *Society, stress and disease*, Volume 1 (pp. 110–124). London: Oxford University Press.

Avons, P., Garthwaite, P., Davies, H.L., Murgatroyd, P.R. & James, W.P.T. (1988). Approaches to estimating physical activity in the community: Calorimetric validation of actometers and heart rate monitoring. *European Journal of Clinical Nutrition*, *42*, 185–196.

Bard, P. (1968). Autonomic nervous system or efferent pathways to visceral effectors. In: V.B. Moutcastle (Ed.), *Medical physiology*, 12th edition, Volume I (pp. 35–68). Saint Louis: Mosby Company.

Barondess, J.A. (1979). Disease and illness – A crucial distinction. *American Journal of Medicine*, *66*, 375–376.

Barry, J., Selwyn, A.P., Nabel, E.G., Rocco, M.B., Mead, K., Campbell, S. & Rebecca, G. (1988). Frequency of ST-segment depression produced by mental stress in stable angina pectoris from coronary artery disease. *American Journal of Cardiology*, *61*, 989–993.

Bartenwerfer, H. (1963). Über Art und Bedeutung der Beziehung zwischen Pulsfrequenz und skalierter psychischer Anspannung. *Zeitschrift für experimentelle und angewandte Psychologie*, *10*, 455–470.

Benzer, A., Niebergall, H., Posch, G. & Flora, G. (1991). Herzfrequenz der Flugretter beim Einsatz im Hubschrauber. *Notfallmedizin*, *17*, 227–232.

Berntson, G.G., Cacioppo, J.T., Binkley, P.F., Uchino, B.N., Quigley, K.S. & Fielstone, A. (1994). Autonomic cardiac control. III. Psychological stress and cardiac response in autonomic space as revealed by pharmacological blockades. *Psychophysiology*, *31*, 599–608.

Bigos, S.J., Battié, M.C., Spengler, D.M., Fisher, L.D., Fordyce, W.E., Hansson, T.H., Nachemson, A.L. & Wortley, M.D. (1991). A prospective study of work perceptions and psychosocial factors affecting the report of back injury. *Spine*, *16*, 1–6.

Blix, A.S., Stromme, S.B. & Ursin, H. (1974). Additional heart rate – an indicator of psychological activation. *Aerospace Medicine*, *45*, 1219–1222.

Böck, D., Rommel, K. & Schröder, R. (1979). Nachfolgeuntersuchung einer Modellvorsorgestudie. *Medizinische Welt*, *30*, 1637–1641.

Bonnet, M.H. & Arand, D.L. (1998). Heart rate variability in insomniacs and matched normal sleepers. *Psychosomatic Medicine*, *60*, 610–615.

Bradley, M.M., Greenwald, M.K. & Hamm, A.O. (1993). Affective picture processing. In: N. Birbaumer & A. Öhman (Eds.), *The structure of emotion* (pp. 48–65). Seattle, WA.: Hogrefe & Huber Publishers.

Brenner, H., Oberacker, A., Kranig, W. & Buchwalsky, R. (1993). A field study on the immediate effects of exposure to low-altitude flights on heart rate and arrhythmia in patients with cardiac diseases. *International Archives of Occupational & Environmental Health*, *65*, 263–268.

Buck, R. (1989). Subjective, expressive, and peripheral bodily components of emotions. In: H. Wagner & A. Manstead (Eds.), *Handbook of social psychophysiology* (pp. 199–221). Chichester: John Wiley & Sons.

Burg, M.M., Jain, D., Soufer, R., Kerns, R.D. & Zaret, B.L. (1993). Role of behavioral and psychological factors in mental stress-induced silent left ventricular dysfunction in coronary artery disease. *Journal of the American College of Cardiology*, *22*, 440–448.

Cabanac, M. (1999). Emotion and phylogeny. *Japanese Journal of Physiology*, *49*, 1–10.

Cacioppo, J.T., Berntson, G.G., Binkley, P.F., Quigley, K.S., Uchino, B.N. & Fielstone, A. (1994). Autonomic cardiac control. II. Noninvasive indices and basal response as revealed by pharmacological blockades. *Psychophysiology*, *31*, 586–598.

Cajochen, C., Pischke, J., Aeschbach, D. & Borbely, A.A. (1994). Heart rate dynamics during human sleep. *Physiology and Behavior*, *55*, 769–774.

Campbell, R.L., Svenson, L.W. & Jarvis, G.K. (1992). Perceived level of stress among university undergraduate students in Edmonton, Canada. *Perceptual and Motor Skills*, *75*, 552–554.

Cannon, W.B. (1929). *Bodily changes in pain, hunger, fear and rage*, 2nd edition (1953). Boston: Charles T. Branford Company.

Cantor, J.R., Zillmann, D. & Bryant, J. (1975). Enhancement of experienced sexual arousal in response to erotic stimuli through misattribution of unrelated residual excitation. *Journal of Personality and Social Psychology*, *32*, 69–75.

Caprara, G.V., D'Imperio, G., Gentilomo, A., Mammucari, A., Renzi, P. & Travaglia, G. (1987). The intrusive commercial: Influence of aggressive TV commercials on aggression. *European Journal of Social Psychology*, *17*, 23–31.

Cline, V.B., Croft, R.G. & Courrier, S. (1973). Desensitization of children to television violence. *Journal of Personality and Social Psychology*, *27*, 360–365.

Cohen , J. (1977). *Statistical power analysis for the behavior sciences*, 2nd edition. New York: Academic Press.

Cohn, P.F. (1989). *Silent myocardial ischemia and infarction.* Basel: Marcel Decker.

Costa, P.T. & McCrae, R.R. (1985). Hypochondriasis, neuroticism, and aging. When are somatic complaints unfounded? *American Psychologist*, *40*, 19–28.

Costa, P.T. & McCrae, R.R. (1987). Neuroticism, somatic complaints, and disease: Is the bark worse than the bite? *Journal of Personality*, *55*, 299–316.

Coulehan, J.L. (1975). Screening yield in an urban low income practice. *American Journal of Public Health*, *65*, 474–479.

Csapo, G. (1980). *Konventionelle und intrakardiale Elektrokardiographie*. Wehr: Ciba-Geigy.

Currie, P. & Saltissi, S. (1993). Transient myocardial ischaemia after acute myocardial infarction does not induce ventricular arrhythmias. *British Heart Journal*, *69*, 303–307.

Deanfield, J.E., Shea, M., Ribiero, P., De Landsheere, C.M., Wilson, R.A., Horlock, P. & Selwyn, A.P. (1984). Transient ST-segment depression as a marker of myocardial ischemia during daily life. *American Journal of Cardiology*, *54*, 1195–1200.

Defoe, D. (1724). *Roxana*. London.

Delle Chiaie, R., Baciarello, G., Villani, M., Iannucci, G., Regine, F., Didonna, A., Talamonti, F. & Pancheri, P. (1996). Cardiovascular reactivity of mitral valve prolapse patients during experimental stress exposure: evidence for a functional nature of cardiovascular symptoms. *Acta Psychiatrica Scandinavica*, *93*, 434–441.

Dimberg, U. (1988). Facial expressions and emotional reactions: a psychobiological analysis of human social behaviour. In: H.L. Wagner (Ed.), *Social psychophysiology and emotion: theory and clinical applications* (pp. 131–150). Chichester: John Wiley & Sons.

Dimberg, U. (1997). Facial reactions: Rapidly evoked emotional responses. *Journal of Psychophysiology*, *11*, 115–123.

Dworkin, S.F. (1991). Illness behavior and dysfunction: review of concepts and application to chronic pain. *Canadian Journal of Physiology and Pharmacology*, *69*, 662–671.

Eggeling, T., Günther, H., Treis-Mueller, I., Osterspey, A., Höher, M. & Hombach, V. (1988). ST-segment changes in healthy volunteers during Holter monitoring and exercise stress test. *European Heart Journal*, *9 (Suppl. N)*, 61–64.

Eisenberg, N., Fabes, R.A., Bustamante, D., Mathy, R.M., Miller, P.A. & Lindholm, E. (1988). Differentiation of vicariously induced emotional reactions in children. *Developmental Psychology*, *24*, 237–246.

Fahrenberg, J. (1994). *Die Freiburger Beschwerdenliste (FBL). Form FBL-G und revidierte Form FBL-R*. Göttingen: Hogrefe.

Fahrenberg, J. (1996). Ambulatory assessment: Issues and perspectives. In: J. Fahrenberg & M. Myrtek (Eds.), *Ambulatory assessment. Computer-assisted psychological and psychophysiological methods in monitoring and field studies* (pp. 3–20). Seattle, WA.: Hogrefe & Huber Publishers.

Fahrenberg, J. & Foerster, F. (1982). Covariation and consistency of activation parameters. *Biological Psychology, 15*, 151–169.

Fahrenberg, J. & Foerster, F. (1991). A multiparameter study in non-invasive cardiovascular assessment. *Journal of Psychophysiology, 5*, 145–158.

Fahrenberg, J., Foerster, F., Schneider, H.J., Müller, W. & Myrtek, M. (1984). *Aktivierungsforschung im Labor-Feld-Vergleich. Zur Vorhersage von Intensität und Mustern psychophysischer Aktivierungsprozesse während wiederholter psychischer und körperlicher Belastung*. München: Minerva.

Fahrenberg, J., Foerster, F., Schneider, H.J., Müller, W. & Myrtek, M. (1985). Adequate scaling of heart rate reactions – A comparative study based on resting levels, measures of basal (sleeping) state, vita maxima, and individual range. In: J.F. Orlebeke, G. Mulder & L.J.P. van Doornen (Eds.), *Psychophysiology of cardiovascular control. Methods, models and data* (pp. 479–490). New York: Plenum.

Fahrenberg, J., Foerster, F., Schneider, H.J., Müller, W. & Myrtek, M. (1986). Predictability of individual differences in activation processes in a field setting based on laboratory measures. *Psychophysiology, 23*, 323–333.

Fahrenberg, J., Franck, M., Baas, U. & Jost, E. (1995). Awareness of blood pressure: interoception or contextual judgement? *Journal of Psychosomatic Research, 39*, 11–18.

Fahrenberg, J., Hampel, R. & Selg, H. (1984). *Das Freiburger Persönlichkeitsinventar FPI.* Göttingen: Hogrefe.

Fahrenberg, J., Leonhart, R. & Foerster, F (2002). *Alltagsnahe Psychologie. Datenerhebung im Feld mit hand-held PC und physiologischem Mess-System.* Bern: Huber.

Fahrenberg, J. & Myrtek, M. (Eds.) (1996). *Ambulatory assessment. Computer-assisted psychological and psychophysiological methods in monitoring and field studies.* Seattle, WA.: Hogrefe & Huber Publishers.

Fahrenberg, J. & Myrtek, M. (Eds.) (2001). *Progress in ambulatory assessment. Computer-assisted psychological and psychophysiological methods in monitoring and field studies.* Seattle, WA.: Hogrefe & Huber Publishers.

Fahrenberg, J., Myrtek, M., Schumacher, J. & Brähler, E. (2000). *Fragebogen zur Lebenszufriedenheit (FLZ). Handanweisung.* Göttingen: Hogrefe.

Fahrenberg, J., Myrtek, M. & Trichtinger, I. (1985). Die Krankheitsursache aus der Sicht des Koronarpatienten. In: W. Langosch (Ed.), *Psychische Bewältigung der chronischen Herzerkrankung* (pp. 32–40). Berlin: Springer.

Fahrenberg, J., Walschburger, P., Foerster, F., Myrtek, M. & Müller, W. (1979). *Psychophysiologische Aktivierungsforschung. Ein Beitrag zu den Grundlagen der multivariaten Emotions- und Stress-Theorie.* München: Minerva.

Fahrenberg, J., Walschburger, P., Foerster, F., Myrtek, M. & Müller, W. (1983). An evaluation of trait, state, and reaction aspects of activation processes. *Psychophysiology, 20*, 188–195.

Falcone, C., Specchia, G., Rondanelli, R., Guasti, L., Corsico, G., Codega, S. & Montemartini, C. (1988). Correlation between beta-endorphin plasma levels and anginal symptoms in patients with coronary artery disease. *Journal of the American College of Cardiology, 11*, 719–723.

Foerster, F. (2001). Assessment of posture, motion, and hand tremor by calibrated accelerometry. In: J. Fahrenberg & M. Myrtek (Eds.), *Progress in ambulatory assessment. Computer-assisted psychological and psychophysiological methods in monitoring and field studies* (pp. 233–256). Seattle, WA.: Hogrefe & Huber Publishers.

Follick, M.J., Ahern, D.K., Gorkin, L., Niaura, R.S., Herd, J.A., Ewart, C., Schron, E.B., Kornfeld, D.S. & Capone, R.J. (1990). Relation of psychosocial and stress reactivity variables to ventricular arrhythmias in the Cardiac Arrhythmia Pilot Study (CAPS). *American Journal of Cardiology*, *66*, 63–67.

Ford, C.V. (1983). *The somatizing disorders – illness as a way of life*. New York: Elsevier.

Frasure-Smith, N. (1987). Levels of somatic awareness in relation to angiographic findings. *Journal of Psychosomatic Research*, *31*, 545–554.

Frauendorf, H. & Kobryn, U. (1975). Richtlinie für die Analyse und Bewertung ausgewählter Formen körperlicher Arbeit. *Zeitschrift für die gesamte Hygiene und ihre Grenzgebiete*, *21*, 21–23.

Freed, C.D., Thomas, S.A., Lynch, J.J., Stein, R. & Friedmann, E. (1989). Blood pressure, heart rate, and heart rhythm changes in patients with heart disease during talking. *Heart & Lung*, *18*, 17–22.

Freeman, L.J. & Nixon, P.G. (1987). Time to rethink the clinical syndrome of angina pectoris? – Implications from ambulatory ST monitoring. *Quarterly Journal of Medicine*, *62*, 25–32.

Freeman, L.J., Nixon, P.G., Sallabank, P. & Reaveley, D. (1987). Psychological stress and silent myocardial ischemia. *American Heart Journal*, *114*, 477–482.

Freud, S. (1940). *Gesammelte Werke*. London: Imago Publishing.

Fridlund, A.J. & Izard, J.T. (1983). Electromyographic studies of facial expressions of emotions and patterns of emotion (pp. 163–218). In: J.T. Cacioppo & R.E. Petty (Eds.), *Social psychophysiology: A source book*. New York: Academic Press.

Frijda, N.H. (1994). Varieties of affect: Emotions and episodes, moods, and sentiments. In: P. Ekman & R.J. Davidson (Eds.), *The nature of emotion. Fundamental questions* (pp. 59–67). New York: Oxford University Press.

Fuller, B.F. (1992). The effects of stress-anxiety and coping styles on heart rate variability. *International Journal of Psychophysiology*, *12*, 81–86.

Gabbay, F.H., Krantz, D.S., Kop, W.J., Hedges, S.M., Klein, J., Gottdiener, J.S. & Rozanski, A. (1996). Triggers of myocardial ischemia during daily life in patients with coronary artery disease: physical and mental activities, anger, and smoking. *Journal of the American College of Cardiology*, *27*, 585–592.

Gottdiener, J.S., Krantz, D.S., Howell, R.H., Hecht, G.M., Klein, J., Falconer, J.J. & Rozanski, A. (1994). Induction of silent myocardial ischemia with mental stress testing: relation to the triggers of ischemia during daily life activities and to ischemic functional severity. *Journal of the American College of Cardiology*, *24*, 1645–1651.

Gray, J.A. (1994). Three fundamental emotion systems. In: P. Ekman & R.J. Davidson (Eds.), *The nature of emotion. Fundamental questions* (pp. 243–247). New York: Oxford University Press.

Gullette, E.C., Blumenthal, J.A., Babyak, M., Jiang, W., Waugh, R.A., Frid, D.J., O'Connor, C.M., Morris, J.J. & Krantz, D.S. (1997). Effects of mental stress on myocardial ischemia during daily life. *Journal of the American Medical Association, 277*, 1521–1526.

Hamburg, D.A., Hamburg, B.A. & Barchas J.D. (1975). Anger and depression in perspective of behavioral biology. In: L. Levi (Ed.), *Emotions – Their parameters and measurement* (pp. 235–278). New York: Raven Press.

Hanratty-Thomas, M.H., Horton, R.W., Lippincott, E.C. & Drabman, R.S. (1977). Desensitization to portrayals of real-life aggression as a function of exposure to television violence. *Journal of Personality and Social Psychology, 35*, 450–458.

Hinz, A., Schreinicke, G. & Hüber, B. (1992). Stability of cardiovascular reactions to mental stressors in repeated studies. *Journal of Psychophysiology, 6*, 155–161.

Hofmann, B., Ladwig, K.H., Schapperer, J., Deisenhofer, I., Marten-Mittag, B., Danner, R. & Schmitt, C. (1999). Psycho-neurogene Faktoren bei der Genese lebensbedrohlicher Arrhythmien. *Nervenarzt, 70*, 830–835.

Hollis, J.F., Connett, J.E., Stevens, V.J. & Greenlick, M.R. (1990). Stressful life events, Type A behavior, and the prediction of cardiovascular and total mortality over six years. MRFIT Group. *Journal of Behavioral Medicine, 13*, 263–280.

Houle, R. & Feldman, R.S. (1991). Emotional displays in children's television programming. *Journal of Nonverbal Behavior, 15*, 261–271.

Jain, D., Burg, M., Soufer, R. & Zaret, B.L. (1995). Prognostic implications of mental stress-induced silent left ventricular dysfunction in patients with stable angina pectoris. *American Journal of Cardiology, 76*, 31–35.

James, W. (1892). *Psychology. The briefer course.* Edited by G. Allport (1985). Notre Dame, IND.: University of Notre Dame Press.

Jäncke, L. (1994). An EMG investigation of the coactivation of facial muscles during the presentation of affect-laden stimuli. *Journal of Psychophysiology, 8*, 1–10.

Jänig, W. (1997). Vegetatives Nervensystem. In: R.F. Schmidt & G. Thews (Eds.), *Physiologie des Menschen*, 27th edition (pp. 340–369). Berlin: Springer.

Jenkins, C.D. (1976). Recent evidence supporting psychologic and social risk factors for coronary disease. *New England Journal of Medicine, 294*, 987–994, 1033–1038.

Johnsen, B.H., Thayer, J.F. & Hugdahl, K. (1995). Affective judgment of the Ekman faces: A dimensional approach. *Journal of Psychophysiology, 9*, 193–202.

Johnson, J.G., Cohen, P., Smailes, E.M., Kasen, S. & Brook, J.S. (2002). Television viewing and aggressive behavior during adolescence and adulthood. *Science, 295*, 2468–2471.

Johnston, D.W. & Anastasiades, P. (1990). The relationship between heart rate and mood in real life. *Journal of Psychosomatic Research, 34*, 21–27.

Jones, G.E., Jones, K.R., Cunningham, R.A. & Caldwell, J.A. (1985). Cardiac awareness in infarct patients and normals. *Psychophysiology, 22*, 480–487.

Kamarck, T.W., Jennings, J.R., Debski, T.T., Glickman-Weiss, E., Johnson, P.S., Eddy, M.J. & Manuck, S.B. (1992). Reliable measures of behaviorally-evoked cardiovascular reactivity from a PC-based test battery: Results from student and community samples. *Psychophysiology, 29*, 17–28.

Käppler, C. & Rieder, S. (2001). Does the retrospection effect hold as a stable phenomenon? – First results from a trans-cultural self-monitoring study of mood and cognitive states in Brazil and Germany. In: J. Fahrenberg & M. Myrtek (Eds.), *Progress in ambulatory assessment. Computer-assisted psychological and psychophysiological methods in monitoring and field studies* (pp. 113–122). Seattle, WA.: Hogrefe & Huber Publishers.

Kasprowics, A., Manuck, S.B., Malkoff, S.B. & Krantz, D.D. (1990). Individual differences in behaviorally evoked cardiovascular response: Temporal stability and hemodynamic patterning. *Psychophysiology, 27*, 605–619.

Katkin, E.S., Morell, M.A., Goldband, S., Bernstein, G.L. & Wise, J.A. (1982). Individual differences in heartbeat discrimination. *Psychophysiology, 19*, 160–166.

Kellner, R. (1991). The significance of somatization *Homeostasis, 33*, 2–6.

Ketterer, M.W. & Buckholtz, C.D. (1989). Somatization disorder. *Journal of the American Osteopathic Association, 89*, 489–490, 495–499.

Kraft, M. & Martin, R.J. (1995). Chronobiology and chronotherapy in medicine. *Disease-A-Month, 41*, 501–575.

Kreutel, K. (1989). *Erfassung des Krankheitsverhaltens. Eine Untersuchung an Herz-Kreislauf-Patienten zu Beginn und am Ende eines stationären Heilverfahrens*. Frankfurt/M.: Peter Lang.

Kuhmann, W., Lachnit, H. & Vaitl, D. (1985). The quantification of experimental load: Methodological and empirical issues. In: A. Steptoe, H. Rüddel & H. Neus (Eds.), *Clinical and methodological issues in cardiovascular psychophysiology* (pp. 45–52). Berlin: Springer.

Kunz, B., Mertens, K. & Oeste, B. (1982). Near-sensor reduction of physiological data by use of a portable microprocessor-system. In: F.D. Stott, E.B. Raftery, D.L. Clement & S.L. Wright (Eds.), *ISAM-Gent-1981* (pp. 464–468). London: Academic Press.

Lacher, D. (1994). *Psychophysiologische Untersuchung zur triadischen Interaktion bei der Diskussion emotional relevanter Themen*. Psychological Institute, University of Freiburg (unpublished thesis).

Lacher, D. (1997). *Partnerschaft im Test. Psychologische und physiologische Untersuchungen an Paaren*. Frankfurt/M.: Peter Lang.

Lang, P.J. (1993). The three-system approach to emotion. In: N. Birbaumer & A. Öhman (Eds.), *The structure of emotion* (pp. 18–30). Seattle, WA.: Hogrefe & Huber Publishers.

Lang, P.J., Davis, M. & Öhman, A. (2000). Fear and anxiety: animal models and human cognitive psychophysiology. *Journal of Affective-Disorders, 61*, 137–159.

LaPorte, R.E., Cauley, J.A., Kinsey, C.M., Corbett, W., Robertson, R., Black-Sandler, R., Kuller, L.H. & Falkel, J. (1982). The epidemiology of physical activity in children, college students, middle-aged men, menopausal females and monkeys. *Journal of Chronic Disease, 35*, 787–795.

LaPorte, R.E., Kuller, L.H., Kupfer, D.J., McPartland, R.J., Matthews, G. & Caspersen, C. (1979). An objective measure of physical activity for epidemiologic research. *American Journal of Epidemiology, 109*, 158–168.

LaPorte, R.E., Montoye, H.J. & Caspersen, C.J. (1985). Assessment of physical activity in epidemiologic research: Problems and prospects. *Public Health Reports*, *100*, 131–46.

Laux, L., Glanzmann, P., Schaffner, P. & Spielberger, C.D. (1981). *Das State-Trait-Angstinventar. Theoretische Grundlagen und Handanweisung*. Weinheim: Beltz.

Leor, J., Poole, W.K. & Kloner, R.A. (1996). Sudden cardiac death triggered by an earthquake. *New England Journal of Medicine*, *334*, 413–419.

Levenson, R.W. (1988). Emotion and the autonomic nervous system: a prospectus for research on autonomic specificity. In: H.L. Wagner (Ed.), *Social psychophysiology and emotion: theory and clinical applications* (pp. 17–42). Chichester: John Wiley & Sons.

Levenson, R.W. (1994). The search for autonomic specificity. In: P. Ekman & R.J. Davidson (Eds.), *The nature of emotion. Fundamental questions* (pp. 252–257). New York: Oxford University Press.

Levick, J.R. (1995). *An introduction to cardiovascular physiology*, 2nd edition. Oxford: Butterworth-Heinemann.

Marshall, J.M. (1968). The heart. In: V.B. Moutcastle (Ed.), *Medical physiology*, 12th edition, Volume I (pp. 35–68). Saint Louis: Mosby Company.

Martinez-Lavin, M., Hermosillo, A.G., Rosas, M. & Soto, M.E. (1998). Circadian studies of autonomic nervous balance in patients with fibromyalgia: a heart rate variability analysis. *Arthritis and Rheumatism*, *41*, 1966–1971.

Mechanic, D. (1962). The concept of illness behavior. *Journal of Chronic Diseases*, *15*, 189–194.

Mechanic, D. & Hansell, S. (1987). Introspection and illness behavior. *Psychiatric Medicine*, *5*, 5–14.

Mellerowicz, H. (1975). *Ergometrie. Grundriß der medizinischen Leistungsmessung*, 2nd edition. München: Urban & Schwarzenberg.

Meshkati, N. (1988). Heart rate variability and mental workload assessment. In: P.A. Hancock & N. Meshkati (Eds.), *Human mental workload* (pp. 101–115). Amsterdam: Elsevier.

Mills, P.J., Berry, C.C., Dimsdale, J.E., Nelesen, R.A. & Ziegler, M.G. (1993). Temporal stability of task-induced cardiovascular, adrenergic, and psychological responses: The effects of race and hypertension. *Psychophysiology*, *30*, 197–204.

Murphy, J.K., Alpert, B.S., Walker, S.S. & Willey, E.S. (1991). Children's cardiovascular reactivity: Stability of racial differences and relation to subsequent blood pressure over a one-year period. *Psychophysiology*, *28*, 447–457.

Musante, L., Treiber, F.A., Kapuku, G., Moore, D., Davis, H. & Strong, W.B. (2000). The effects of life events on cardiovascular reactivity to behavioral stressors as a function of socioeconomic status, ethnicity, and sex. *Psychosomatic Medicine*, *62*, 760–767.

Myrtek, M. (1975). Fehlerkoeffizienten bei klinisch-physiologischen Messungen und klinisch-chemischen Analysen. *Medizinische Welt*, *26*, 2144–2149.

Myrtek, M. (1984). *Constitutional psychophysiology: Research in review*. Orlando, FLA.: Academic Press.

Myrtek, M. (1985). Adaptation effects and stability coefficients of repeated testing for rest, strain, and change scores. In: A. Steptoe, H. Rüddel & H. Neus (Eds.), *Clinical and methodological issues in cardiovascular psychophysiology* (pp. 72–105). Berlin: Springer.

Myrtek, M. (1990). Covariation and reliability of ECG parameters during 24-hour monitoring. *International Journal of Psychophysiology, 10*, 117–123.

Myrtek, M. (1997). Streß und Typ-A-Verhalten. In: P. Allhoff, G. Flatten & U. Laaser (Eds.), *Krankheitsverhütung und Früherkennung. Handbuch der Prävention*, 2nd edition (pp. 315–336). Berlin: Springer.

Myrtek, M. (1998a). *Gesunde Kranke – kranke Gesunde. Psychophysiologie des Krankheitsverhaltens*. Bern: Huber.

Myrtek, M. (1998b). Metaanalysen zur Psychophysiologischen Persönlichkeitsforschung. In: F. Rösler (Ed.), *Enzyklopädie der Psychologie. Themenbereich C, Theorie und Forschung. Serie I, Biologische Psychologie, Band 5: Ergebnisse und Anwendungen der Psychophysiologie* (pp. 285–344). Göttingen: Hogrefe.

Myrtek, M. (2000). *Das Typ-A-Verhaltensmuster und Hostility als eigenständige Risikofaktoren der koronaren Herzkrankheit.* (Reihe Statuskonferenz Psychokardiologie, Eds.: J. Jordan, B. Bardé & A.M. Zeiher. Band 2). Frankfurt/M.: Verlag für Akademische Schriften.

Myrtek M. (2001). Subjektive Beschwerden und objektiver Schweregrad bei Herzerkrankungen. In: B. Rauch & K. Held (Eds.), *Der schwerkranke und multimorbide Herzpatient. Eine Herausforderung für die kardiologische Rehabilitation* (pp. 149–153). Darmstadt: Steinkopff.

Myrtek, M. (2002). Psychophysiologische Untersuchungen zum gestörten Schlaf. In: M. Myrtek (Ed.), *Die Person im biologischen und sozialen Kontext* (pp. 61–83). Göttingen: Hogrefe.

Myrtek, M. & Brügner, G. (1996). Perception of emotions in everyday life: studies with patients and normals. *Biological Psychology, 42*, 147–164.

Myrtek, M., Brügner, G. & Fichtler, A. (1990). Diurnal variations of ECG parameters during 23-hour-monitoring in cardiac patients with ventricular arrhythmias or ischemic episodes. *Psychophysiology, 27*, 620–626.

Myrtek, M., Brügner, G., Fichtler, A., König, K., Müller, W., Foerster, F. & Höppner V. (1988). Detection of emotionally induced ECG changes and their behavioral correlates: A new method for ambulatory monitoring. *European Heart Journal, 9 (Suppl. N)*, 55–60.

Myrtek, M., Brügner, G., Fichtler, A. & Müller, W. (1994). Testretest stability of ECG parameters during ambulatory monitoring of patients with ischemic heart disease. *Journal of Ambulatory Monitoring, 7*, 265–279.

Myrtek, M., Brügner, G. & Müller, W. (1996a). Interactive monitoring and contingency analysis of emotionally induced ECG changes: Methodology and applications. In: J. Fahrenberg & M. Myrtek (Eds.), *Ambulatory assessment. Computer-assisted psychological and psychophysiological methods in monitoring and field studies* (pp. 115–127). Seattle, WA.: Hogrefe & Huber Publishers.

Myrtek, M., Brügner, G. & Müller, W. (1996b). Validation studies of emotional, mental, and physical workload components in the field. In: J. Fahrenberg & M. Myrtek (Eds.), *Ambu-*

latory assessment. Computer-assisted psychological and psychophysiological methods in monitoring and field studies (pp. 287–304). Seattle, WA.: Hogrefe & Huber Publishers.

Myrtek, M., Deutschmann-Janicke, E., Strohmaier, H., Zimmermann, W., Lawerenz, S., Brügner, G. & Müller, W. (1994). Physical, mental, emotional, and subjective workload components in train drivers. *Ergonomics*, *37*, 1195–1203.

Myrtek, M., Dieterle, W. & Brügner, G. (1990). Psychophysiological response patterns to variations of the experimental load of a reaction time task. *Journal of Psychophysiology*, *4*, 209–220.

Myrtek, M., Fichtler, A., König, K., Brügner, G. & Müller, W. (1994). Differences between patients with asymptomatic and symptomatic myocardial infarction: The relevance of psychological factors. *European Heart Journal*, *15*, 311–317.

Myrtek, M., Fichtler, A., Strittmatter, M. & Brügner, G. (1999). Stress and strain of blue and white collar workers during work and leisure time: Results of psychophysiological and behavioral monitoring. *Applied Ergonomics*, *30*, 341–351.

Myrtek, M. & Foerster, F. (2001). On-line measurement of additional heart rate. Methodology and applications. In: J. Fahrenberg & M. Myrtek (Eds.), *Progress in ambulatory assessment. Computer-assisted psychological and psychophysiological methods in monitoring and field studies* (pp. 399–414). Seattle, WA.: Hogrefe & Huber Publishers.

Myrtek, M. & Foerster, F. (in press). Freiburg monitoring system (FMS). In: G.R.J. Hockey, A.W.K. Gaillard & O. Burov (Eds.), *Operator functional state: The assessment and prediction of human performance degradation in complex tasks*. Amsterdam: IOS Press.

Myrtek, M. Foerster, F. & Brügner, G. (2001). *Freiburger Monitoring System (FMS). Ein Daten-Aufnahme- und Auswertungs-System für Untersuchungen im Alltag: Emotionale Beanspruchung, Körperlage, Bewegung, EKG, subjektives Befinden, Verhalten*. Frankfurt/M.: Peter Lang.

Myrtek, M., Frölich, E., Fichtler, A. & Brügner, G. (2000). ECG changes, emotional arousal, and subjective state. An ambulatory monitoring study with CHD patients. *Journal of Psychophysiology*, *14*, 106–114.

Myrtek, M., Hilgenberg, B., Brügner, G. & Müller W. (1997). Influence of sex, college major, and chronic study stress on psychophysiological reactivity and behavior: Results of ambulatory monitoring in students. *Journal of Psychophysiology*, *11*, 124–137.

Myrtek, M., Itte, H., Zimmermann, W. & Brügner, G. (1994). Psychische Bewältigung von Unfällen bei Lokomotivführern: Die Relevanz von Copingfragebogen zur Erfassung von funktionalen und dysfunktionalen Copingprozessen. *Zeitschrift für Klinische Psychologie*, *23*, 293–304.

Myrtek, M. & Nahrwold, A. (1974). Zur Vorhersage der körperlichen Leistungsfähigkeit. Schätzung der maximalen Sauerstoffaufnahme aus submaximalen Messwerten und anthropometrischen Daten. *Herz/Kreislauf*, *6*, 194–199.

Myrtek, M. & Scharff, C. (2000). *Fernsehen, Schule und Verhalten. Untersuchungen zur emotionalen Beanspruchung von Schülern*. Bern: Huber.

Myrtek, M. & Spital, S. (1986). Psychophysiological response patterns to single, double, and triple stressors. *Psychophysiology*, *23*, 663–671.

Myrtek, M., Zanda, D. & Aschenbrenner, E. (2001). Interactive psychophysiological monitoring of emotions in students' everyday life. A replication study. In: J. Fahrenberg & M. Myrtek (Eds.), *Progress in ambulatory assessment. Computer-assisted psychological and psychophysiological methods in monitoring and field studies* (pp. 415–434). Seattle, WA.: Hogrefe & Huber Publishers.

Nerell, G. & Wahlund, I. (1981). Stressors and strain in white collar workers. In: L. Levi (Ed.), *Society, stress and disease, Vol 4, Working life* (pp. 120–127). Oxford: Oxford University Press.

Otzenberger, H., Gronfier, C., Simon, C., Charloux, A., Ehrhart, J., Piquard, F. & Brandenberger, G. (1998). Dynamic heart rate variability: a tool for exploring sympathovagal balance continuously during sleep in men. *American Journal of Physiology, 275*, H946–H950.

Parkinson, B. (1988). Arousal as a cause of emotion. In: H.L. Wagner (Ed.), *Social psychophysiology and emotion: theory and clinical applications* (pp. 85–104). Chichester: John Wiley & Sons.

Pennebaker, J.W. (1982). *The psychology of physical symptoms*. New York: Springer.

Pennebaker, J.W. & Hoover, C.W. (1984). Visceral perception versus visceral detection: Disentangling methods and assumptions. *Biofeedback and Self Regulation, 9*, 339–352.

Piech, R. (2002). *Achterbahn und Autobahn. Psychophysiologisches Monitoring zum Freizeitstress*. Psychological Institute, University of Freiburg (unpublished thesis).

Pivik, R.T. & Busby, K. (1996). Heart rate associated with sleep onset in preadolescents. *Journal of Sleep Research, 5*, 33–36.

Pivik, R.T., Busby, K.A., Gill, E., Hunter, P. & Nevins, R. (1996). Heart rate variations during sleep in preadolescents. *Sleep, 19*, 117–135.

Plutchik, R. (2003). *Emotions and life. Perspectives from psychology, biology, and evolution*. Washington, DC.: American Psychological Association.

Pringle, S.D., Macfarlane, P.W. & Cobbe, S.M. (1989). Response of heart rate to a roller coaster ride. *British Medical Journal, 299*, 1575.

Quyyumi, A.A., Crake, T., Wright, C., Mockus, L., Levy, R.D. & Fox, K.M. (1986). The incidence and morphology of ischaemic ventricular tachycardia. *European Heart Journal, 7*, 1037–1044.

Rahe, R.H. (1974). Life change and subsequent illness reports. In: E.K.E. Gunderson & R.H. Rahe (Eds.), *Life stress and illness* (pp. 58–78). Springfield, ILL.: Thomas.

Rehman, A., Zalos, G., Andrews, N.P., Mulcahy, D. & Quyyumi, A.A. (1997). Blood pressure changes during transient myocardial ischemia: insights into mechanisms. *Journal of the American College of Cardiology, 30*, 1249–1255.

Reisenzein, R. (1983). The Schachter theory of emotion: Two decades later. *Psychological Bulletin, 94*, 239–264.

Rimé, B., Philippot, P. & Cisamolo, D. (1990). Social schemata of peripheral changes in emotion. *Journal of Personality and Social Psychology, 59*, 38–49.

Ring, C. & Brener, J. (1996). Influence of beliefs about heart rate and actual heart rate on heartbeat counting. *Psychophysiology, 33*, 541–546.

Ring, C., Liu, X. & Brener, J. (1994). Cardiac stimulus intensity and heartbeat detection: effects of tilt-induced changes in stroke volume. *Psychophysiology*, *31*, 553–564.

Rissanen, V., Romo, M. & Siltanen, P. (1978). Premonitory symptoms and stress factors preceding sudden death from ischaemic heart disease. *Acta Medica Scandinavica*, *204*, 389–396.

Robra, B.P., van der Heyden, E. & Machens, D. (1982). Herz-Kreislauf-Vorsorgeprogramm VW/Salzgitter. Auswertung der Ergebnisse 1974 bis 1979. *Niedersächsisches Ärzteblatt*, *21*, 757–766.

Roge, J., Pebayle, T. & Muzet, A. (2001).Variations of the level of vigilance and of behavioural activities during simulated automobile driving. *Accident Analysis and Prevention*, *33*, 181–186.

Rohmert, W. & Rutenfranz, J. (1975). *Arbeitswissenschaftliche Beurteilung der Belastung und Beanspruchung an unterschiedlichen industriellen Arbeitsplätzen.* Bonn: Der Bundesminister für Arbeit und Sozialordnung (Ed.), Referat Öffentlichkeitsarbeit.

Rommel, K., Steinhardt, B. & Überla, K. (1976). Modell-Vorsorgeuntersuchung in zwei Betrieben. *Klinische Wochenschrift*, *54*, 1169–1175, 1177–1185, 1187–1192.

Roth, D.L., Bachtler, S.D. & Fillingim, R.B. (1990). Acute emotional and cardiovascular effects of stressful mental work during aerobic exercise. *Psychophysiology*, *27*, 694–701.

SAS Institute (1993). *SAS Procedures Guide, Version 6*. Cary, NC.: SAS Institute.

Sausen, K.P., Lovallo, W.R., Pincomb, G.A. & Wilson, M.F. (1992). Cardiovascular responses to occupational stress in male medical students: A paradigm for ambulatory monitoring studies. *Health Psychology*, *11*, 55–60.

Schachter, S. & Singer, J. (1962). Cognitive, social, and physiological determinants of emotional state. *Psychological Review*, *69*, 379–399.

Schandry, R. (1981). Heart beat perception and emotional experience. *Psychophysiology*, *18*, 483–488.

Schandry, R., Bestler, M. & Montoya, P. (1993). On the relation between cardiodynamics and heartbeat perception. *Psychophysiology*, *30*, 467–474.

Scherer, K.R. (1990). Theorien und aktuelle Probleme der Emotionspsychologie. In: K.R. Scherer (Ed.), *Enzyklopädie der Psychologie, Themenbereich C, Serie IV, Band 3: Psychologie der Emotion* (pp. 1–38). Göttingen: Hogrefe.

Scherer, K.R. (2000). Psychological models of emotion. In: J.C. Borod (Ed.), *The neuropsychology of emotion* (pp.137–162). Oxford: Oxford University Press.

Schwaberger, G. (1987). Heart rate, metabolic and hormonal responses to maximal psycho-emotional and physical stress in motor car racing drivers. *International Archives of Occupational and Environmental Health*, *59*, 579–604.

Schwartz, J.E., Warren, K. & Pickering, T.G. (1994). Mood, location, and physical position as predictors of ambulatory blood pressure and heart rate: Application of a multi-level random effects model. *Annals of Behavioral Medicine*, *16*, 210–220.

Schwarzer, R. (1989). *Meta-analysis programs*. Berlin: Institute of Psychology (http://user page.fu-berlin.de/~health/meta_e.htm).

Schwenkmezger, P., Hodapp, V. & Spielberger, C.D. (1992). *Das State-Trait-Ärgerausdrucks-Inventar STAXI*. Bern: Huber.

Selye, H. (1950). *The physiology and pathology of exposure to stress*. Montreal: Acta.

Selye, H. (1956). *The stress of life*, 8th edition. New York: McGraw Hill.

Selye, H. (1976). *Stress in health and disease. Chapter I: History and general outline of the stress concept* (pp. 3–34). Boston: Butterworth.

Shapiro, D., Jamner, L.D. & Goldstein, I.B. (1997). Daily mood states and ambulatory blood pressure. *Pychophysiology, 34*, 399–405.

Shapiro, D., Jamner, L.D., Lane, J.D., Light, K.C., Myrtek, M., Sawada, Y. & Steptoe, A. (1996). Blood pressure publication guidelines. *Psychophysiology, 33*, 1–12.

Shear, M.K., Kligfield, P., Harshfield, G., Devereux, R.B., Polan, J.J., Mann, J.J., Pickering, T. & Frances, A.J. (1987). Cardiac rate and rhythm in panic patients. *American Journal of Psychiatry, 144*, 633–637.

Sloan, E.P., Natarajan, M., Baker, B., Dorian, P., Mironov, D., Barr, A., Newman, D.M. & Shapiro, C.M. (1999). Nocturnal and daytime panic attacks – comparison of sleep architecture, heart rate variability, and response to sodium lactate challenge. *Biological Psychiatry, 45*, 1313–1320.

Stemmler, G. (1989). The autonomic differentiation of emotions revisited: Convergent and discriminant validation. *Psychophysiology, 26*, 617–632.

Stemmler, G. & Fahrenberg, J. (1989). Psychophysiological assessment: Conceptual, psychometric, and statistical issues. In: G. Turpin (Ed.), *Handbook of Clinical Psychology* (pp. 71–103). Chichester: John Wiley & Sons.

Stephan, E., Mutz, G., Feist, A. & Weiss, R.K. (2001). Some new developments in ambulatory assessment devices. In: J. Fahrenberg & M. Myrtek (Eds.), *Progress in ambulatory assessment. Computer-assisted psychological and psychophysiological methods in monitoring and field studies* (pp. 561–568). Seattle, WA.: Hogrefe & Huber Publishers.

Stern, S., Gavish, A., Weisz, G., Benhorin, J., Keren, A. & Tzivoni, D. (1988). Characteristics of silent and symptomatic myocardial ischemia during daily activities. *American Journal of Cardiology, 61*, 1223–1228.

Strasser, H. (1982). *Arbeitswissenschaftliche Methoden der Beanspruchungsermittlung*. Schriftenreihe Arbeitsmedizin, Sozialmedizin, Präventivmedizin, Band 69. Stuttgart: Gentner.

Taggart, P., Gibbons, D. & Somerville, W. (1969). Some effects of motorcar driving on the normal and abnormal heart. *British Medical Journal, 4*, 130–134.

Taylor, E.W., Jordan, D. & Coote, J.H. (1999). Central control of the cardiovascular and respiratory systems and their interactions in vertebrates. *Physiological Reviews, 79*, 855–916.

Theorell, T., Lind, E. & Floderus, B. (1975). The relationship of disturbing life-changes and emotions to the early development of myocardial infarction and other serious illnesses. *International Journal of Epidemiology, 4*, 281–293.

Thomas, S.A., Freed, C.D., Friedmann, E., Stein, R., Lynch, J.J. & Rosch, P.J. (1992). Cardiovascular responses of patients with cardiac disease to talking and exercise stress testing. *Heart Lung*, *21*, 64–73.

Tryon, W.W. (1991). *Activity measurement in psychology and medicine*. New York: Plenum.

Turner, J.R., Carroll, D., Hanson, J. & Sims, J. (1988). A comparison of additional heart rates during active psychological challenge calculated from upper body and lower body dynamic exercise. *Psychophysiology*, *25*, 209–216.

Uexküll, T. von (1963). *Grundfragen der psychosomatischen Medizin*. Reinbek: Rowohlt Verlag.

Van de Borne, P., Biston, P., Paiva, M., Nguyen, H., Linkowski, P. & Degaute, J.P. (1995). Cardiorespiratory transfer during sleep: a study in healthy young men. *American Journal of Physiology*, *269 (3 Pt 2)*, H952–H958.

Watson, D. & Pennebaker, J.W. (1989). Health complaints, stress, and distress: Exploring the central role of negative affectivity. *Psychological Review*, *96*, 234–254.

Weitkunat, R., Schandry, R., Sparrer, B. & Beck, K. (1987). Zur Trainierbarkeit der Herzwahrnehmung. *Zeitschrift für Experimentelle und Angewandte Psychololologie*, *34*, 340–350.

Wilhelm, P., Myrtek, M. & Brügner, G. (1997). *Vorschulkinder vor dem Fernseher. Ein psychophysiologisches Feldexperiment*. Bern: Huber.

Wilson, B.J. (1991). Children's reactions to dreams conveyed in mass media programming. *Communication Research*, *18*, 283–305.

Wilson, G.F. (1988). Measurement of operator workload with the neuropsychological workload test battery. In: P.A. Hancock & N. Meshkati (Eds.), *Human mental workload* (pp. 63–100). Amsterdam: Elsevier.

Wilson, G.F. (2001). In-flight psychophysiological monitoring. In: J. Fahrenberg & M. Myrtek (Eds.), *Progress in ambulatory assessment. Computer-assisted psychological and psychophysiological methods in monitoring and field studies* (pp. 435–454). Seattle, WA.: Hogrefe & Huber Publishers.

Windmann, S., Schonecke, O.W., Fröhlig, G. & Maldenar, G. (1999). Dissociating beliefs about heart rates and actual heart rates in patients with cardiac pacemakers. *Psychophysiology*, *36*, 339–342.

Wink, K., Bödicker, U. & Kaufmann, B. (1983). Der Stellenwert der Prodromi beim akuten Myokardinfarkt. *Therapiewoche*, *33*, 4741–4746.

World Health Organization (1967). *Manual of the international statistical classification of diseases, injuries, and causes of death*, Volume 1. Geneva: WHO.

World Health Organization (1977). *Manual of the international statistical classification of diseases, injuries, and causes of death*, Volume 1. Geneva: WHO.

World Health Organization (1992). *International statistical classification of diseases and related health problems, ICD-10*, Volume 1. Geneva: WHO.

Wundt, W. (1905). *Grundzüge der physiologischen Psychologie*. Leipzig: Engelmann.

Yeragani, V.K., Sobolewski, E., Igel, G., Johnson, C., Jampala, V.C., Kay, J., Hillman, N., Yeragani, S. & Vempati, S. (1998). Decreased heart-period variability in patients with panic disorder: a study of Holter ECG records. *Psychiatry Research, 78*, 89–99.

Zanda, D. (1999). *Le emozioni catturate. Un monitoraggio delle emozioni quotidiane di studenti universitari.* Facolta di Psicologia, Padua (unpublished thesis).

Zemaityte, D., Varoneckas, G. & Sokolov, E. (1984). Heart rhythm control during sleep. *Psychophysiology, 21*, 279–289.

Zillmann, D. & Bryant, J. (1982). Pornography, sexual callousness, and the trivialization of rape. *Journal of Communication, 32*, 10–21.

Zillmann, D. & Bryant, J. (1988). Pornography's impact on sexual satisfaction. *Journal of Applied Social Psychology, 18*, 438–453.

Authors index

Subject index

F

G

H

I

J

L

M